CLINICAL CASE PRESENTATIONS

FOR

VETERINARY HEMATOLOGY

AND CLINICAL CHEMISTRY

CLINICAL CASE PRESENTATIONS

FOR

VETERINARY HEMATOLOGY

AND CLINICAL CHEMISTRY

Mary Anna Thrall, D.V.M., M.S., D.A.C.V.P.
Professor, Department of Microbiology, Immunology,
and Pathology
College of Veterinary Medicine and Biomedical Sciences
Colorado State University
Fort Collins, Colorado

Dale C. Baker, D.V.M., Ph.D., D.A.C.V.P.
Pathologist, Genentech, Inc.
South San Francisco, California

Terry W. Campbell, D.V.M., Ph.D.
Professor, Department of Clinical Sciences
College of Veterinary Medicine and Biomedical Sciences
Fort Collins, Colorado

Dennis DeNicola, D.V.M., Ph.D., D.A.C.V.P.
Chief Veterinary Educator
IDEXX Laboratories
North Grafton, Massachusetts

Martin J. Fettman, D.V.M., M.S., Ph.D., D.A.C.V.P.
Associate Dean, College of Veterinary Medicine and
Biomedical Sciences
Colorado State University
Fort Collins, Colorado

E. Duane Lassen, D.V.M., Ph.D., D.A.C.V.P.
Professor, Department of Microbiology, Immunology,
and Pathology
College of Veterinary Medicine and Biomedical Sciences
Colorado State University
Fort Collins, Colorado

Alan Rebar, D.V.M., Ph.D., D.A.C.V.P.
Dean, School of Veterinary Medicine
Purdue University
West Lafayette, Indiana

Glade Weiser, D.V.M., D.A.C.V.P.
Vice President, Diagnostics/Clinical Pathologist
Heska Corporation
Fort Collins, Colorado

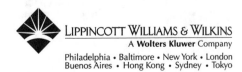
LIPPINCOTT WILLIAMS & WILKINS
A **Wolters Kluwer** Company
Philadelphia • Baltimore • New York • London
Buenos Aires • Hong Kong • Sydney • Tokyo

Editor: David B. Troy
Managing Editor: Rebecca A. Kerins
Marketing Manager: Samantha S. Smith
Production Editor: Jennifer D. W. Glazer
Designer: Doug Smock
Compositor: Circle Graphics
Printer: RR Donnelley

Library of Congress Cataloging-in-Publication Data
Clinical case presentations for veterinary hematology and clinical chemistry / Mary Anna
    Thrall ... [et al.].
        p. ; cm.
    Includes index.
    ISBN 0-7817-5799-1
        1. Veterinary hematology—Case studies. 2. Veterinary clinical chemistry—Case studies.
    I. Thrall, Mary Anna. II. Veterinary hematology and clinical chemistry.
    [DNLM: 1. Hematologic Diseases—veterinary—Case Reports. 2. Clinical Chemistry
    Tests—methods—Case Reports. 3. Hematologic Diseases—diagnosis—Case Reports. 4.
    Laboratory Techniques and Procedures—veterinary—Case Reports. SF 769.5 C641 2004]
    SF769.5.C63 2004
    636.089'615—dc22

                                                                    2004044162

04 05 06 07 08
1 2 3 4 5 6 7 8 9 10

The authors wish to dedicate this book to their mentors, the pioneers in veterinary clinical pathology. In particular, the book is dedicated to Drs. Maxine Benjamin, Oscar Schalm, and J. J. Kaneko for their respective first-generation textbooks addressing veterinary clinical pathology, hematology, and clinical chemistry, and their inspiration to many subsequent careers in veterinary clinical pathology. Mary Anna Thrall also wishes to thank Dr. Maxine Benjamin for her generosity, patience, and friendship.

CONTENTS

HEMATOLOGY

Case 1	2	Case 6	9
Case 2	4	Case 7	10
Case 3	6	Case 8	11
Case 4	7	Case 9	12
Case 5	8	Case 10	13

COAGULATION

Case 11	15	Case 13	18
Case 12	17	Case 14	19

RENAL

Case 15	21	Case 21	34
Case 16	23	Case 22	37
Case 17	25	Case 23	39
Case 18	27	Case 24	40
Case 19	30	Case 25	41
Case 20	32	Case 26	43

GASTROINTESTINAL FLUID AND ELECTROLYTE

Case 27	44	Case 30	50
Case 28	46	Case 31	52
Case 29	48		

HEPATIC

Case 32	53	**Case 38**	65
Case 33	55	**Case 39**	67
Case 34	57	**Case 40**	69
Case 35	59	**Case 41**	70
Case 36	61	**Case 42**	71
Case 37	62	**Case 43**	72

PANCREAS

Case 44	74	**Case 45**	76

GLUCOSE METABOLISM

Case 46	78	**Case 47**	80

ENDOCRINE

Case 48	82	**Case 53**	91
Case 49	83	**Case 54**	93
Case 50	85	**Case 55**	95
Case 51	87	**Case 56**	97
Case 52	89	**Case 57**	99

CASE DISCUSSIONS

This book presents a number of case studies taken from animal medical records. Each case is presented with its relevant clinicopathologic data. The cases are organized more or less by the primary disease or organ system involved in disease, realizing that many of them have multiple system abnormalities. In addition to the first 10 cases focusing on hematology, examples of hematologic disease are dispersed throughout the remaining series of cases.

Interpretation of laboratory data is an art that is developed through accumulated experience. The interactions and patterns of data related to disease diagnosis are complex. One also must develop an appreciation for magnitudes of abnormality that influence interpretation of each measurement. This case discussion appendix is designed to provide the reader both experience and guidance in beginning to learn the art of interpretation. This art is then continually cultivated through real-time experience in the clinical setting.

The laboratory data are presented for each case in a form that allows the reader to learn from making their own effort at describing and interpreting data. Please note the following formatting:

1. Data are presented in conventional units. In some areas, international (SI) units are given; these are shown in italics.
2. Laboratory values that are abnormal and central to the interpretation are given in bold type.

Following each data set, an interpretive discussion is presented. These narratives may be used by the reader for self-assessment of proficiency in interpretation of data.

The following terms may be abbreviated throughout the case discussions.

aPTT	Activated partial thromboplastin time
ALT	Alanine aminotransferase
Alb	Albumin
ALP	Alkaline phosphatase
An. gap	Anion gap
AST	Aspartate aminotransferase
Bands	Band Neutrophils
BUN	Blood urea nitrogen
Ca	Calcium
Calc. Osmolality	Calculated osmolality
CL	Chloride
Chol	Cholesterol
CK	Creatine Kinase
Creat	Creatinine
Eos	Eosinophils
Epith cells	Epithelial cells
GGT	Gamma glutamyl transferase
Glob	Globulin
Gluc	Glucose
Hgb	Hemoglobin
hpf	High power field
K	Potassium
lpf	Low power field
Lymphs	Lymphocytes
MCV	Mean cell volume
MCHC	Mean corpuscular hemoglobin concentration
Meas. Osmolality	Measured osmolality
Metas	Metamyelocytes
Monos	Monocytes
Na	Sodium
NCC	Total nucleated cell count
NRBCs	Nucleated Red blood cells
PCV	Packed cell volume
Phos	Phosphorus
PT	Prothrombin time
RBC	Red blood cell
Retics	Reticulocytes
SDH	Sorbitol dehydrogenase
Segs	Segmented neutrophils
Sp. gr.	Specific gravity
T. Bili	Total bilirubin
TCO_2	Total CO_2
TP	Total protein
TP (P)	Total plasma protein
TP (S)	Total serum protein
WBCs	White blood cells

CASE 1

Signalment and History: 11-year-old male cat. Lethargy and polydipsia. One month ago PCV was 38%.

Hematology		Reference Range
PCV (%)	13	25–45
RBC (×10⁶/µl)	1.55	5–11
Hgb (g/dl)	4.0	8–15
MCV (fl)	84	39–50
MCHC (g/dl)	31	33–37
Retics (/µl)	155,000	0–60,000
NCC (×10³/µl)	20.6	5.5–19.5
Metas (×10³/µl)	0.4	0
Bands (×10³/µl)	0.8	0–0.3
Segs (×10³/µl)	9.9	2.5–12.5
Lymphs (×10³/µl)	1.4	1.5–7.0
Monos (×10³/µl)	3.1	0–0.8
Eos (×10³/µl)	0.2	0–1.5
Nucleated RBCs (×10³/µl)	4.8	0
Platelets (×10³/µl)	Adequate	150–700
TP (P) (g/dl)	8.9	6.0–8.5

Hemopathology: Many *Hemobartonella felis* (*Mycoplasma haemofelis*) organisms on erythrocytes. Occasional reactive lymphocyte.

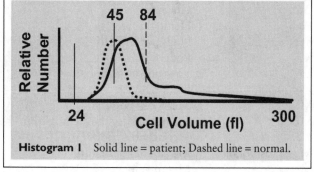

Histogram 1   Solid line = patient; Dashed line = normal.

Biochemical Profile		Reference Range
Gluc (mg/dl)	249	67–124
BUN (mg/dl)	96	17–32
Creat (mg/dl)	6.6	0.9–2.1
Ca (mg/dl)	10.2	8.5–11
Phos (mg/dl)	7.9	3.3–7.8
TP (g/dl)	8.4	5.9–8.1
Alb (g/dl)	3.3	2.3–3.9
Glob (g/dl)	5.1	2.9–4.4
T. Bili (mg/dl)	0.3	0–0.3
Chol (mg/dl)	386	60–220
ALT (IU/L)	53	30–100
ALP (IU/L)	19	6–106
Na (mEq/L)	150	146–160
K (mEq/L)	4.9	3.7–5.4
CL (mEq/L)	127	112–129
TCO₂ (mEq/L)	10	14–23
An. gap (mEq/L)	18	10–27
Calc. osmolality (mOsm/kg)	337	290–310

Urinalysis (cystocentesis)			
Color	Yellow	**Urine Sediment**	
Transparency	Cloudy	WBCs/hpf	6–8
Sp. gr.	1.020	RBCs/hpf	1–2
Protein	Negative	Epith cells/hpf	1–3 transitional
Gluc	2+	Casts/lpf	0
Bilirubin	Negative	Crystals	0
Blood	Negative	Bacteria	0
pH	5.0	Other	fat
Ketones	Negative		

Interpretive Discussion

Hematology

Packed cell volume, Hemoglobin, Red blood cell count: The cat is anemic; all measurements of red blood cell mass are decreased.

MCV: The mean cell volume is increased, which one would expect with a regenerative anemia. However, the increase is greater than can be accounted for by the reticulocytes, suggesting that agglutination is causing the increase, since doublets are being counted as one erythrocyte. This is confirmed by the histogram.

Reticulocytes are increased, indicating that the anemia is regenerative. Regenerative anemia is due to blood loss or blood destruction.

Nucleated RBCs are increased due to early marrow release, and are often present in a regenerative anemia.

Erythrocyte morphology: The presence of *Hemobartonella felis* (*Mycoplasma haemofelis*) organisms explains the anemia (blood destruction). Agglutination is likely due to the presence of antibodies against the organisms.

Monocytosis and increased immature (band) neutrophils are indicative of an inflammatory leukogram.

Lymphopenia is indicative of a stress or inflammatory leukogram.

Total protein: Total protein is increased. In this patient, it is due to hyperglobulinemia (see biochemical profile interpretation below).

Biochemical Profile

The serum glucose concentration is moderately increased. This could be due to stress (glucocorticoid release), as the lymphopenia suggests, but could also be due to diabetes mellitus.

The BUN and serum creatinine concentrations are increased, and in the face of a urine specific gravity of only 1.020, is indicative of renal azotemia.

The serum phosphorus concentration is mildly increased, and is compatible with decreased glomerular filtration rate.

The serum total protein concentration is increased due to an increase in the globulin concentration. The increase in globulin should trigger protein electrophoresis to determine if gammopathy is monoclonal or polyclonal.

The serum cholesterol concentration is moderately increased. This may be due to metabolic disorders associated with diabetes mellitus.

Serum total CO_2 is decreased, suggesting metabolic acidosis.

The increased calculated serum osmolality is primarily due to hyperglycemia and increased BUN.

Urinalysis

As evidenced by the low urine specific gravity in the face of azotemia, the animal is not concentrating adequately, indicating renal dysfunction. The presence of glucose indicates that the renal threshold of glucose has been exceeded.

Summary

This animal had been previously diagnosed with diabetes mellitus and was not being controlled adequately. *Hemobartonella felis* (*Mycoplasma haemofelis*) is often an opportunist in cats that are immunosuppressed. The hyperglobulinemia was polyclonal, indicating antigenic stimulation, possibly due to *Hemobartonella felis*.

CASE 2

Signalment: 5-year-old spayed female cocker spaniel
History: Acutely lethargic
Physical Examination: Pale, slightly icteric, mucous membranes

Hematology		Reference Range
PCV (%)	**12**	37–55
Hgb (g/dl)	**3.6**	12–18
RBC (×10⁶/µl)	**0.95**	5.5–8.5
MCV (fl)	**114**	60–72
MCHC (g/dl)	30	34–38
Retics (/µl)	**123**	<60
NCC (×10³/µl)	**96.1**	6–17
Segs (×10³/µl)	**69.1**	3–11.5
Bands (×10³/µl)	**6.7**	0–0.3
Metas (×10³/µl)	**1.0**	0
Monos (×10³/µl)	**5.8**	0.1–1.3
Lymphs (×10³/µl)	**0**	1–4.8
Eos (×10³/µl)	0	0.1–1.2
NRBCs (×10³/µl)	**13.5**	0
Platelets (×10³/µl)	284	200–500
TP (P) (g/dl)	6.8	6–8

Hemopathology: Polychromasia increased, agglutination present, many spherocytes present. Occasional Howell-Jolly body.

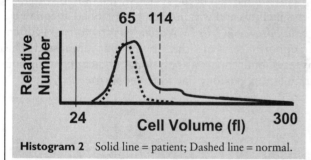

Histogram 2   Solid line = patient; Dashed line = normal.

Biochemical Profile		Reference Range
Gluc (mg/dl)	**143**	75–130
BUN (mg/dl)	**39**	7–28
Creat (mg/dl)	1.3	0.9–1.7
Ca (mg/dl)	9.0	9.0–11.2
Phos (mg/dl)	4.4	2.8–6.1
TP (g/dl)	6.5	5.4–7.4
Alb (g/dl)	3.3	2.7–4.5
Glob (g/dl)	3.2	1.9–3.4
T. Bili (mg/dl)	**4.7**	0–0.4
Chol (mg/dl)	269	130–370
ALT/µl (IU/L)	32	10–120
AST/µl (IU/L)	30	16–40
ALP (IU/L)	**438**	35–280
Na (mEq/L)	146	145–158
K (mEq/L)	5.0	4.1–5.5
CL (mEq/L)	118	106–127
TCO₂ (mEq/L)	14	14–27
An. gap (mEq/L)	19	8–25

Urinalysis (catheterized)			
Color	Orange	**Urine Sediment**	
Transparency	Turbid	WBCs/hpf	0
Sp. Gr.	1.038	RBCs/hpf	**10**
Protein	1+	Epith cells/hpf	0
Gluc	Negative	Casts/lpf	0
Bilirubin	**2+**	Crystals	Numerous **Bilirubin**
Blood	**1+**	Bacteria	0
pH	6.0		

Interpretive Discussion

Hematology

Packed cell volume, Hemoglobin, Red blood cell count: The dog is very anemic, as all measurement of red blood cells mass are decreased. The RBC count is likely erroneously decreased, due to erythrocyte agglutination, and groups of red blood cells being counted as one red blood cell.

MCV: The mean cell volume is erroneously increased due to agglutination. Although the anemia is regenerative, the MCV is much higher than can be accounted for by an increase in reticulocytes. As one can see on the histogram, erythrocytes that are agglutinated are being counted as one large erythrocyte.

Reticulocytes are increased, indicating that the anemia is regenerative, suggesting either blood loss or blood destruction.

Nucleated RBCs are increased, likely due to early release from bone marrow in response to marked anemia. However, it is also possible that the dog has decreased splenic function secondary to glucocorticosteroid administration.

Erythrocyte morphology: Presence of spherocytes and agglutination, in the absence of a previous blood transfusion, are indicative of immune mediated hemolytic anemia.

Neutrophilia, increased immature neutrophils, and monocytosis are indicative of a markedly inflammatory leukogram. The absence of lymphocytes is suggestive of stress or corticosteroids. Inflammatory leukograms are commonly seen in association with immune mediated hemolytic anemia.

Biochemical Profile

Glucose is mildly increased. Considering the lymphopenia, this may be due to stress or steroids.

BUN is increased, suggesting decreased GFR or bleeding into the GI tract. Since the creatinine is within the reference range, and the dog is concentrating urine, this is likely prerenal azotemia, due to GI hemorrhage (high protein diet) or decreased blood flow to the kidneys.

Bilirubin is increased, indicating either cholestasis or increased red blood cell destruction. Because the dog has immune mediated hemolytic anemia, increased RBC destruction is most likely.

Serum alkaline phosphatase activity is increased, which could be due to either cholestasis or previous treatment with corticosteroids.

Urinalysis

Bilirubinuria and the presence of bilirubin crystals reflect the increased serum bilirubin concentration. Conjugated bilirubin readily passes through glomeruli and is then excreted in the urine. Blood and protein may be present due to traumatic catheterization. The animal is concentrating, indicating that the increase in BUN is not due to renal dysfunction.

Summary

This is a typical case of immune mediated hemolytic anemia. Dog was treated with prednisone and recovered. It had been previously treated with corticosteroids, accounting for the stress leukogram, hyperglycemia, and increased serum alkaline phosphatase activity.

CASE 3

Signalment and History: 11-year-old DSH spayed female cat presented for anorexia and lethargy.

Hematology		Reference Range
PCV (%)	13	25–45
RBC (×10⁶/µl)	1.84	5–11
Hgb (g/dl)	4.2	8–15
MCV (fl)	71	39–50
MCHC (g/dl)	32	33–37
Retics (/µl)	7,360	0–60,000
Nucleated cells (×10³/µl)	71.3	5.5–19.5
Metas (×10³/µl)	0.7	0
Bands (×10³/µl)	2.1	0–0.3
Segs (×10³/µl)	33.2	2.5–12.5
Lymphs (×10³/µl)	2.8	1.5–7.0
Monos (×10³/µl)	6.9	0–0.8
NRBCs (×10³/µl)	24.9	0
Blasts (×10³/µl)	0.7	0
Platelets (×10³/µl)	Adequate	150–700
TP (P) (g/dl)	8.0	6.0–8.5

Hemopathology: Blasts appear to be rubriblasts. Many prorubricytes and rubricytes also present.

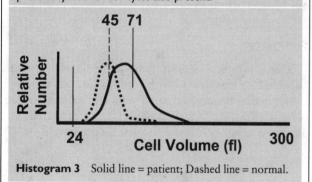

Histogram 3   Solid line = patient; Dashed line = normal.

Interpretive Discussion

Hematology

Packed cell volume, Hemoglobin, Red blood cell count: Cat is markedly anemic. Reticulocytes are not increased, indicating that the anemia is nonregenerative.

MCV is markedly increased, in the absence of reticulocytosis or agglutination. In a cat, this should trigger testing for feline leukemia virus, as the MCV may be increased as a result of viral-induced erythrodysplasia. Macrocytosis with widened histogram is often seen in FeLV positive cats with anemia.

Neutrophilia, increased band neutrophils and metamyelocytes, and monocytosis are indicative of inflammation.

Nucleated red blood cells are increased in the absence of reticulocytes. Moreover, many of these are quite immature, indicating that the cat has leukemia involving the erythrocytes.

Summary

Myeloproliferative disorder, erythremic myelosis or M6(E).

CASE 4

Signalment and History: 17-year-old male cat presented for lethargy and enlarged abdomen. Liver disease suspected, but biochemical profile normal.

Hematology		Reference Range
PCV (%)	24	25–45
MCV (fl)	33	39–50
MCHC (g/dl)	32	33–37
Retics (/µl)	ND	0–60,000
Nucleated cells (×10³/µl)	13.2	5.5–19.5
Bands (×10³/µl)	4.5	0–0.3
Segs (×10³/µl)	6.6	2.5–12.5
Lymphs (×10³/µl)	0.5	1.5–7.0
Monos (×10³/µl)	0.5	0–0.8
Eos (×10³/µl)	0.3	0–1.5
Basophils (×10³/µl)	0.8	rare
Platelets (×10³/µl)	Adequate	150–700
TP (P) (g/dl)	6.6	6.0–8.5

Hemopathology: Many keratocytes, schistocytes.

Histogram 4   Solid line = patient; Dashed line = normal.

Interpretive Discussion

Hematology

Packed cell volume: The cat is mildly anemic.

MCV: The mean cell volume is decreased. Decreased mean cell volume is almost always caused by iron deficiency anemia, which in adults is almost always secondary to chronic blood loss.

Erythrocyte morphology: Keratocytes are commonly associated with iron deficiency anemia. Iron deficiency anemia is not as common in cats as in dogs, and the few cases we have seen did not have increased central pallor.

The total leukocyte count and the mature neutrophil concentration are within the reference range, but the increase in band neutrophils is indicative of inflammation. Lymphopenia is suggestive of a stress or previous corticosteroid administration.

Total protein is within the reference range. Although one might expect total protein to be decreased with chronic blood loss, animals often compensate for this chronic loss of protein.

Summary

Owner declined further diagnostic evaluation. Chronic GI blood loss secondary to an intestinal tumor would be the most likely diagnosis in this aged patient with iron deficiency anemia.

CASE 5

Signalment: 1-year-old pointer

History: Treated for neck or back pain with corticosteroids by referring veterinarian. Dog was thought to have GI parasites due to occult blood in feces, and was treated with anthelmintics. The dog returned 1 month later with a PCV of 15% and MCV of 40 fl. At that time the dog had an abdominal effusion.

Physical Examination: Painful abdomen, pale mucous membranes

Hematology		Reference Range
PCV (%)	**18**	37–55
Hgb (g/dl)	3.76	12–18
RBC (×10⁶/µl)	5.8	5.5–8.5
MCV (fl)	**47**	60–72
MCHC (g/dl)	33	34–38
Retics (/µl)	**18**	<60
NCC (×10³/µl)	**40.1**	6–17
Segs (×10³/µl)	**36.5**	3–11.5
Bands (×10³/µl)	**0.4**	0–0.3
Metas (×10³/µl)	**0.4**	0
Monos (×10³/µl)	1.2	0.1–1.3
Lymphs (×10³/µl)	1.2	1–4.8
Eos (×10³/µl)	0.4	0.1–1.2
Platelets (×10³/µl)	**623**	200–500
TP (P) (g/dl)	5.9	6–8

Hemopathology: Numerous keratocytes, few schistocytes, some RBCs appear hypochromic. Occasional lymphocyte with azurophilic granules.

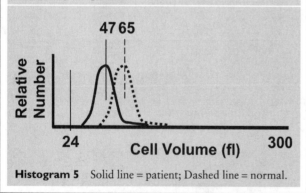

Histogram 5   Solid line = patient; Dashed line = normal.

Abdominal Fluid Analysis		
NCC (µl)	90,000	
TP (g/dl)	4.0	

Cytology: All cells are degenerate neutrophils. Bacteria of various types are present.

Interpretive Discussion

Hematology

Packed cell volume, Hemoglobin: Both are decreased, indicating that the dog is anemic. The red blood cell count is within the reference range, suggesting erythrocytes are small.

MCV: The mean cell volume is decreased. Decreased mean cell volume is almost always caused by iron deficiency anemia, which in adults is almost always secondary to chronic blood loss.

Reticulocytes are not increased, indicating that the anemia is nonregenerative. While uncomplicated iron deficiency anemia is usually regenerative, this anemia may be nonregenerative due to the presence of inflammation (note inflammatory leukogram).

Erythrocyte morphology: Keratocytes, erythrocyte fragmentation, and increased central pallor are commonly associated with iron deficiency anemia.

Neutrophilia and increased immature neutrophils are indicative of a markedly inflammatory leukogram. The inflammatory leukogram is compatible with the presence of inflammation in the peritoneal cavity, although one would usually expect to see more band neutrophils in dogs with peritonitis. The presence of this inflammation may be the explanation for the lack of a regenerative response to the anemia, as an anemia of inflammatory disease may be superimposed on the iron deficiency anemia.

Platelets are increased. Approximately half of all animals with iron deficiency anemia have increased platelets, probably in response to cytokines and growth factors.

Total protein: Total protein is slightly decreased, probably as a result of chronic blood loss.

Histogram confirms the presence of a population of microcytic cells (normal histogram represented by dashed line).

Abdominal Fluid Analysis

Suppurative septic inflammation. The presence of different types of bacteria suggests a GI source of bacteria.

Summary

The dog died, and on necropsy had an intestinal perforation secondary to an ulcer, chronic diffuse peritonitis, pyogranulomatous lymphadenitis and amyloidosis of the spleen, liver, and kidney. Presumably, the dog had been chronically bleeding from this ulcer, resulting in iron deficiency anemia.

CASE 6

Signalment and History: 9 year-old female Beagle presented for lethargy and pale mucous membranes. Owner reported that the dog occasionally had blood in feces.

Hematology		Reference Range
PCV (%)	12	37–55
RBC (×10⁶/µl)	2.76	5.5–8.5
Hgb (g/dl)	3.2	12–18
MCV (fl)	40	60–72
MCHC (g/dl)	29	34–38
Retics (/µl)	242,880	0–60,000
Nucleated cells (×10³/µl)	33.4	6.0–17.0
Metas (×10³/µl)	–	0
Bands (×10³/µl)	–	0–0.3
Segs (×10³/µl)	30.7	3.0–11.5
Lymphs (×10³/µl)	1.0	1.0–4.8
Monos (×10³/µl)	1.0	0.2–1.4
Eos (×10³/µl)	–	0.1–1.2
NRBCs (×10³/µl)	0.7	0
Platelets (×10³/µl)	Adequate	200–500
TP (P) (g/dl)	6.3	6.0–8.0

Hemopathology: Increased central pallor, occasional keratocyte, giant platelets.

Interpretive Discussion

Hematology

Packed cell volume, Hemoglobin, Red blood cell count: The dog is markedly anemic; all measurements of red blood cell mass are decreased.

MCV: The mean cell volume is markedly decreased. Decreased mean cell volume is almost always caused by iron deficiency anemia, which in adults is almost always secondary to chronic blood loss.

Reticulocytes are increased, indicating that the anemia is regenerative, suggesting blood loss or blood destruction. In this case, the decreased MCV strongly suggests iron deficiency anemia secondary to chronic blood loss. The presence of nucleated red blood cells is compatible with this degree of regenerative response.

Erythrocyte morphology: Keratocytes and increased central pallor are commonly associated with iron deficiency anemia.

Neutrophilia is indicative of inflammation, even though no band neutrophils are present, since the neutrophil concentration is greater than two fold upper reference range. The lymphocyte count is in the low normal range, indicating that there may be a stress or steroid component to the neutrophilia.

Total protein is within the reference range. Although one might expect total protein to be decreased with chronic blood loss, animals often compensate for this chronic loss of protein.

Summary

GI barium series performed and jejunal mass seen. At surgery, mass in mid-jejunum resected, determined to be a leiomyosarcoma with clean surgical margins. The regenerative response in this case is in contrast to the previous case to make the point that iron deficiency anemia may be either regenerative or nonregenerative.

CASE 7

Signalment: 10-year-old castrated male Labrador retriever

History: Four episodes of acute weakness over past 3 months. At time of wellness exam 4 months ago, dog had PCV of 44% and T.P. of 8.2 g/dl.

Physical Examination: Pale mucous membranes, abdomen slightly distended.

Hematology		Reference Range
PCV (%)	**16**	37–55
Hgb (g/dl)	**5.3**	12–18
RBC (×10⁶/µl)	**2.48**	5.5–8.5
MCV (fl)	63	60–72
MCHC (g/dl)	34	34–38
Retics (/µl)	**342**	<60
NCC (×10³/µl)	**39.1**	6–17
Segs (×10³/µl)	**33.2**	3–11.5
Bands (×10³/µl)	**1.2**	0–0.3
Monos (×10³/µl)	**3.1**	0.1–1.3
Lymphs (×10³/µl)	**0.4**	1–4.8
Eos (×10³/µl)	0.4	0.1–1.2
NRBCs (×10³/µl)	0.8	0
Platelets (×10³/µl)	**130**	200–500
TP (P) (g/dl)	6.2	6–8

Hemopathology: Polychromasia increased, numerous acanthocytes and schistocytes. Numerous Howell-Jolly bodies

Biochemical Profile		
No abnormalities		

Abdominal Fluid Analysis		
PCV (%)	24%	
NCC (/µl)	34,000	

Cytology: 95% nondegenerate neutrophils; 5% macrophages, many of which have phagocytized erythrocytes

Interpretive Discussion

Hematology

Packed cell volume, Hemoglobin, Red blood cell count: The dog is anemic; all measurements of red blood cell mass are decreased.

MCV: The mean cell volume is normal. However, it is surprising that it is not higher considering that the reticulocyte count is increased

Reticulocytes are increased, indicating that the anemia is regenerative, and is thus due to blood loss or blood destruction.

Nucleated RBCs are increased due to early marrow release.

Erythrocyte morphology: Acanthocytes are commonly seen in dogs with hemangiosarcoma. The schistocytes are suggestive of microangiopathy, which may also be associated with hemangiosarcoma.

Neutrophilia, increased immature (band) neutrophils, and monocytosis are indicative of an inflammatory leukogram, although a component of the mature neutrophilia is likely due to stress or corticosteroids.

Lymphopenia is indicative of a stress or steroid leukogram.

Platelets are slightly decreased. Considering the presence of schistocytes, the animal may have DIC.

Total protein: Total protein is within the reference range. However, considering that it was 8.2 g/dl 4 months previously, it is likely decreased due to blood loss within the abdominal cavity.

Abdominal Fluid Analysis

Hemoabdomen

Summary

The signalment (large breed, older dog), history (episodes of weakness), regenerative anemia, erythrocyte morphology, and the hemoabdomen are all suggestive of hemangiosarcoma. An exploratory was performed, and the dog had hemangiosarcoma of the spleen and liver, which had ruptured. Previous episodes of weakness were likely due to previous ruptures of the tumor, which had subsequently sealed, then ruptured again.

CASE 8

Signalment: 15-year-old Staffordshire terrier
History: Lethargic
Physical Examination: Pale mucous membranes

Hematology	January	October	Reference Range
PCV (%)	30	28	37–55
RBC (×10⁶/µl)	4.70	4.44	5.5–8.5
Hgb (g/dl)	10.1	9.5	12–18
MCV (fl)	61	64	60–72
MCHC (g/dl)	35	34	34–38
Retics (/µl)	178,000	13,200	0–60,000
NCC (×10³/µl)	23.4	10.2	6.0–17.0
Bands (×10³/µl)	0.5	0.2	0–0.3
Segs (×10³/µl)	15.7	6.2	3.0–11.5
Lymphs (×10³/µl)	6.1	1.5	1.0–4.8
Monos (×10³/µl)	0.7	1.7	0.2–1.4
Eos (×10³/µl)	–		0.1–1.2
NRBCs (×10³/µl)	–		0
Platelets (×10³/µl)	150	12	200–500
TP (g/dl)	8.2	5.6	6.0–8.0
Alb	1.5		2.7–4.5
Glob	6.0		1.9–3.4

Hemopathology (January): Increased rouleaux, giant platelets, lymphs contain azurophilic granules.
Hemopathology (October): Increased rouleaux, lymphs contain azurophilic granules. numerous *Hemobartonella canis* (*Mycoplasma haemocanis*) organisms present.

Interpretive Discussion

Hematology

Packed cell volume, Hemoglobin, Red blood cell count: The dog is anemic; all measurements of red blood cell mass are decreased.

Reticulocytes are increased in January, indicating that the anemia is regenerative, suggesting either blood loss or blood destruction. Although the PCV is further decreased in October, the anemia is no longer regenerative, suggesting bone marrow dysfunction.

Monocytosis and increased immature (band) neutrophils are indicative of an inflammatory leukogram (January).

Lymphocytosis in January is most suggestive of either lymphocytic leukemia or ehrlichiosis.

Platelets: The animal is markedly thrombocytopenic in October. The combination of thrombocytopenia and nonregenerative anemia should trigger a bone marrow aspirate examination and ehrlichia titer. Common causes of thrombocytopenia include ehrlichiosis, immune mediated thrombocytopenia, and DIC.

Total protein: Total protein is increased. In this patient, it is due to hyperglobulinemia, which should trigger protein electrophoresis.

The presence of increased rouleaux is compatible with increased globulin. The presence of large granular lymphocytes is suggestive of certain types of antigenic stimulation, commonly ehrlichiosis, or a leukemia of LGL cells. The presence of *Hemobartonella canis* (*Mycoplasma hemocanis*) organisms in October suggests either a previous splenectomy or splenic dysfunction, since the erythrocyte parasite is rarely seen in dogs with functional spleens. The anemia is no longer regenerative in the face of this erythrocyte parasite, suggesting marrow impairment of some type, and a bone marrow aspirate is indicated.

Summary

In January, the anemia was possibly due to blood loss associated with a large hematoma of the spleen, and the dog was splenectomized. The lymphocytosis, hyperglobulinemia, and presence of large granular lymphocytes should have triggered an ehrlichia titer, but did not. The animal returned in October, severely anemic and thrombocytopenic. An ehrlichia titer was done at this time, and was strongly positive. The dog was treated for ehrlichiosis and hemobartonellosis, and recovered.

CASE 9

Signalment and History: 9-year-old male castrated dog presented for lethargy.

Hematology		Reference Range
PCV (%)	36	37–55
RBC (×10⁶/μl)	5.42	5.5–8.5
Hgb (g/dl)	13.2	12–18
MCV (fl)	66	60–72
MCHC (g/dl)	37	34–38
Retics (/μl)	0	0–60,000
NCC (×10³/μl)	96.4	6.0–17.0
Metas (×10³/μl)	–	0
Bands (×10³/μl)	7.7	0–0.3
Segs (×10³/μl)	82.9	3.0–11.5
Lymphs (×10³/μl)	1.0	1.0–4.8
Monos (×10³/μl)	4.8	0.2–1.4
Eos (×10³/μl)	–	0.1–1.2
NRBCs (×10³/μl)	–	0
Platelets (×10³/μl)	39	200–500
TP (P) (g/dl)	6.2	6.0–8.0

Hemopathology: Decreased platelets, giant platelets, toxic neutrophils, numerous echinocytes, occasional schistocyte,

Interpretive Discussion

Hematology

Packed cell volume and hemoglobin are slightly decreased, indicating mild anemia.

Reticulocytes are not increased, indicating that the anemia is nonregenerative. Considering the inflammatory leukogram, this is most likely an anemia of inflammatory disease.

Marked neutrophilia with increased immature neutrophils and monocytosis is indicative of an inflammatory leukogram.

Lymphopenia is indicative of a stress or steroid leukogram.

Platelets are decreased. Thrombocytopenia is most commonly due to ehrlichiosis, immune mediated thrombocytopenia or DIC. This should trigger other coagulation tests. The presence of giant platelets suggests that immature platelets are being released by the bone marrow, and the thrombocytopenia is not due to bone marrow dysfunction.

Summary

Anemia of inflammatory disease. Site of inflammation was a prostatic abscess. DIC was confirmed.

CASE 10

Signalment: 4-year-old Doberman
History: Acutely ill, vomiting
Physical Examination: Pendulous abdomen

Hematology	Day 1*	Day 2	Reference Range
PCV (%)	50	20	37–55
Hgb (g/dl)	18.3	7.5	12–18
RBC (×10⁶/µl)	7.70	3.11	5.5–8.5
MCV (fl)	66	66	60–72
MCHC (g/dl)	36	37	34–38
Retics (/µl)	ND	124	<60
NCC (×10³/µl)	6.6	14.7	6–17
Segs (×10³/µl)	0.4	4.1	3–11.5
Bands (×10³/µl)	3.1	7.9	0–0.3
Metas (×10³/µl)	0.1	1.5	0
Monos (×10³/µl)	0.5	0.3	0.1–1.3
Lymphs (×10³/µl)	2.1	0.4	1–4.8
Eos (×10³/µl)	0.1	0.1	0.1–1.2
Platelets (×10³/µl)	193	90	200–500
TP (P) (g/dl)	5.9	4.0	6–8

Hemopathology: neutrophils on Days 1 and 2.

* Had abdominal exploratory surgery the evening of Day 1; treated with fluids between Day 1 and Day 2

Biochemical Profile	Day 1*	Day 2	Reference Range
Gluc	26	36	75–130
BUN (mg/dl)	45	62	7–28
Creat (mg/dl)	0.6	1.8	0.9–1.7
Ca (mg/dl)	8.2	7.6	9.0–11.2
Phos (mg/dl)	5.9	11.0	2.8–6.1
TP (g/dl)	4.5	2.6	5.4–7.4
Alb (g/dl)	1.8	1.0	2.7–4.5
Glob (g/dl)	2.7	1.0	1.9–3.4
T. Bili (mg/dl)	0.1	3.0	0–0.4
Chol (mg/dl)	145	140	130–370
ALT (IU/L)	20	328	10–120
AST (IU/L)	77	775	16–40
ALP (IU/L)	208	440	35–280
GGT	1	1	0–6
Na (mEq/L)	136	143	145–158
K (mEq/L)	4.1	5.8	4.1–5.5
CL (mEq/L)	100	106	106–127
TCO₂ (mEq/L)	9.4	19.4	14–27
An. gap (mEq/L)	31	23	8–25

* Had abdominal exploratory surgery the evening of Day 1; treated with fluids between Day 1 and Day 2

Abdominal Fluid Analysis	
NCC (/µl)	93,000
TP (g/dl)	1.5

Cytology: 100% degenerate neutrophils; various types of bacteria phagocytized and free.

Interpretive Discussion

Hematology

Packed cell volume, Hemoglobin, Red blood cell count: Within or near reference range on Day 1, markedly decreased on Day 2 following blood loss that occurred at the time of surgery. Dog seemed to bleed excessively during the surgery.

Reticulocytes are increased on Day 2, indicating that the anemia is regenerative. This regenerative response is earlier than is typically seen, in that reticulocytes don't usually increase until 24 to 72 hours following the onset of anemia.

Neutropenia is present on Day 1, with an increase in immature neutrophils, indicating in this case that the mature neutrophils are being consumed in an inflammatory process, and the marrow is not keeping up with the demand. This type of response is commonly referred to as a degenerative left shift. On Day 2, the mature neutrophils have increased, as have the immature neutrophils (bands and metamyelocytes). This indicates that the consumptive process has decreased (source of inflammation) or that the marrow has increased production, or both.

Lymphopenia is indicative of a stress or steroid leukogram.

Platelets are mildly decreased on Day 1, and more markedly decreased on Day 2. While some platelets may have been consumed in clotting process secondary to surgery related blood loss, it is also possible that the animal has DIC, particularly with the history of excessive bleeding during surgery. This should trigger additional tests such as FDPs, PT, APTT, and activated clotting time.

Total protein: Total protein is decreased on Day 1 and Day 2. In this patient, this is likely due to loss into the abdominal cavity on Day 1, compounded by blood loss on Day 2. Fluid administration may also be diluting the PCV and plasma protein on Day 2.

Biochemical Profile

The serum glucose concentration is markedly decreased, both on Day 1 and Day 2. In this patient, considering the leukogram, this is most likely due to sepsis. Other differentials should include insulinoma, although this is a relatively young dog for an insulinoma.

The BUN is increased on both Day 1 and Day 2, and the serum creatinine is increased on Day 2. This may be either prerenal azotemia or renal azotemia. A urinalysis was not performed.

The serum calcium is decreased on both Days 1 and 2, and is due to the hypoalbuminemia.

The serum phosphorus concentration is increased on Day 2 and is compatible with decreased glomerular filtration rate.

The serum total protein concentration is decreased due to hypoalbuminemia on Day 1, and both hypoalbuminemia and hypoglobulinemia on Day 2 (see explanation above).

The serum bilirubin concentration is increased on Day 2, likely due to cholestasis related to septicemia.

The ALT and AST activity is increased on Day 2, possibly related to anemia, shock, surgery, or septicemia.

The ALP activity is increased on Day 2, possibly related to endogenous corticosteroids or cholestasis.

Both sodium and chloride are decreased on Day 1, possibly due to loss of electrolytes into abdominal effusion, or loss due to vomiting.

Serum total CO_2 is decreased on Day 1, suggesting metabolic acidosis. This has been corrected by Day 2, likely due to fluid therapy.

The anion gap is increased on Day 1, likely due to lactic acid.

Abdominal Fluid

The nucleated cell count is very high and all of the cells present are neutrophils, indicating suppurative inflammation. The total protein may be low because the serum protein is decreased, or it may be diluted in the large volume of fluid. The presence of different types of bacteria suggests that the source of bacteria is the gastrointestinal tract.

Summary

This dog had a degenerative left shift and hypoglycemia due to sepsis. On exploratory, the abdominal cavity contained 1400 ml of fluid, and a toothpick was found to have perforated the intestine. Dog died on the evening of Day 2 as a result of septic peritonitis.

CASE 11

Signalment: 8-year-old spayed female golden retriever
History: Presented for lethargy, anorexia, a mass over the humeroradial joint, and prolonged bleeding at a biopsy site.
Physical Examination: There was fever, icterus, and an enlarged liver and spleen.

Hematology		Reference Range
PCV (%)	23	37–55
Hgb (g/dl)	8.5	12–18
RBC (×10⁶/µl)	3.27	5.5–8.5
MCV (fl)	71	60–72
MCHC (g/dl)	37	34–38
Retics (/µl)	130.8	< 60
NCC (×10³/µl)	45.4	6–17
Segs (×10³/µl)	41.8	3–11.5
Bands (×10³/µl)	0.5	0–0.3
Monos (×10³/µl)	3.2	0.1–1.3
Lymphs (×10³/µl)	0.0	1–4.8
Eos (×10³/µl)	0.0	0.1–1.2
Platelets (×10³/µl)	25	200–500
TP (P) (g/dl)	4.6	6–8
Hemopathology: Increased polychromasia and giant platelets		

Biochemical Profile		Reference Range
Gluc (mg/dl)	70	65–122
BUN (mg/dl)	11	7–28
Ca (mg/dl)	8.2	9.0–11.2
Phos (mg/dl)	4.0	2.8–6.1
TP (g/dl)	5.0	5.4–7.4
Alb (g/dl)	2.2	2.7–4.5
Glob (g/dl)	2.8	1.9–3.4
T. Bili (mg/dl)	7.6	0–0.4
Chol (mg/dl)	329	130–370
ALT (IU/L)	58	10–120
ALP (IU/L)	775	35–280
Na (mEq/L)	144	145–158
K (mEq/L)	4.0	4.1–5.5
CL (mEq/L)	109	106–127
TCO₂ (mEq/L)	16.6	14–27
An. gap (mEq/L)	22	8–25

Urinalysis			
Color	Yellow	**Urine Sediment**	
Transparency	Clear	WBCs/hpf	0–2
Sp. Gr.	1.012	RBCs/hpf	0–1
Protein	–	Epith cells/hpf	0
Gluc	–	Casts/lpf	0
Bilirubin	4+	Crystals	0
Blood	Trace	Bacteria	0
pH	5.5	Other	1+fat

Coagulation Data		Reference Range
Activated clotting time (seconds)	>300	72–86
PT (seconds)	14.5	6.4–7.4
aPTT (seconds)	32.3	9–11
FDPs (µg/ml)	>80	<10

Interpretative Discussion

Hematology

There is anemia that is regenerative as evidenced by the significant reticulocytosis and polychromasia. Anemia in combination with low total protein suggests that the cause is external blood loss; however, low albumin in conjunction with normal globulin suggests decreased production or loss of albumin, rather than blood loss, as the cause of hypoproteinemia. There is a mixed inflammatory and stress (steroid) leukogram evidenced by the neutrophilia with band neutrophils, monocytosis, and absence of lymphocytes and eosinophils. The thrombocytopenia in conjunction with the large platelets suggests increased consumption and production of platelets.

Biochemical Profile

Hypocalcemia corrects into the normal range, and thus is due to hypoalbuminemia. Hypoproteinemia is due primarily to hypoalbuminemia. Since there is no significant proteinuria, hypoproteinuria may be due to loss through the intestinal tract or lack of production by the liver. Starvation may also cause hypoalbuminemia. The hyperbilirubinemia may result from increased erythrocyte destruction or cholestasis. Increased alkaline phosphatase activity supports cholestasis. Very mild hyponatremia and hyperkalemia are probably insignificant in this case.

Urinalysis

The urine specific gravity is isosthenuric, but the urea nitrogen is normal, so the specific gravity may not be significant. Water deprivation and ensuing specific gravity would determine renal function. Hyperbilirubinuria is a consequence of hyperbilirubinemia.

Coagulation Data

Decreased platelets, prolonged ACT, PT, aPTT, and increased FDPs support disseminated intravascular coagulation. Erythrocytes may be destroyed during disseminated intravascular coagulation, thus contributing to elevated total bilirubin.

Summary

The mass was diagnosed as malignant histiocytosis, with nodules in the liver, spleen, mediastinum, and peripheral lymph nodes at necropsy. A likely scenario is that extensive tumor mass developed necrosis and/or inflammation that triggered hypercoagulability leading to disseminated intravascular coagulation. Involvement of liver likely explains the hypoalbuminemia and other liver changes.

CASE 12

Signalment: 5-month-old female dog

History: The puppy bleeds excessively when it loses teeth.

Physical Examination: The mucous membranes were pale. There is moderate bleeding evident at the site of a recent tooth loss.

Hematology		Reference Range
PCV (%)	19	37–55
Hgb (g/dl)	6.1	12–18
Retics (/µl)	188	< 60
NCC (×10³/µl)	35.4	6–17
Segs (×10³/µl)	29.7	3–11.5
Bands (×10³/µl)	2.5	0–0.3
Monos (×10³/µl)	3.2	0.1–1.3
Lymphs (×10³/µl)	0.0	1–4.8
Eos (×10³/µl)	0.0	0.1–1.2
Platelets (×10³/µl)	915	200–500
TP (P) (g/dl)	6.5	6–8

Hemopathology: Moderate polychromasia and anisocytosis is present.

Coagulation Data		Reference Range
Activated clotting time	>180	72–86
PT (seconds)	6.8	6.4–7.4
aPTT (seconds)	>120	9–11
Fibrinogen (mg/dl)	200	100–400
Bleeding Time (minutes)	3	1–5

Interpretative Discussion

Hematology

The anemia is regenerative as the reticulocyte count is increased and there is polychromasia and anisocytosis on the blood film. The cause of anemia is not determined, but is likely due to hemolysis or blood loss since it is regenerative. The clinical findings of hemorrhage suggest that blood loss is the cause. Thrombocytosis is common in iron deficiency anemia. Microcytosis is evident in chronic iron deficiency, and may contribute to anisocytosis. Size of erythrocytes is not known, since the MCV is not provided. Serum iron and iron binding capacity would be useful in determination of the cause of anemia. The neutrophilia, left shift, and monocytosis indicate an inflammatory leukogram. Lymphopenia is indicative of a stress/steroid mediated response.

Coagulation Data

The coagulation profile suggests a deficiency of one or multiple coagulation factors in the intrinsic pathway. Platelet concentration is increased in number, and no large forms are seen in peripheral blood. Bleeding time is normal, and in the face of normal platelet concentration, indicates that platelet function is normal. The most common cause of a severe coagulopathy with normal platelet concentration, normal hepatic enzyme activity, and a prolongation of the aPTT with normal PT is factor 8 deficiency. The occurrence is less common in females, and to have an affected female requires that the sire also be affected.

Summary

This dog was tested for factor 8 plasma activity and was found to have 21% of normal activity, which is diagnostic for factor 8 deficiency or hemophilia A. This is compatible with the major abnormalities in the ACT and APTT and the clinical description of bleeding in a young dog.

CASE 13

Signalment: 7-year-old female Walker Hound

History: The owner noticed a swelling on the right front leg on the day of admission.

Physical Examination: The mucous membranes were pale. There was a subcutaneous swelling in the right ventral thoracic area, with some dried blood on all four legs.

Hematology		Reference Range
PCV (%)	**25**	37–55
Hgb (g/dl)	**8.4**	12–18
RBC (×10⁶/μl)	**4.03**	5.5–8.5
MCV (fl)	62	60–72
MCHC (g/dl)	34	34–38
Retics (/μl)	44	< 60
NCC (×10³/μl)	14.4	6–17
Segs (×10³/μl)	**12.2**	3–11.5
Monos (×10³/μl)	**1.6**	0.1–1.3
Lymphs (×10³/μl)	**0.6**	1–4.8
Platelets (×10³/μl)	315	200–500
TP (P) (g/dl)	**4.6**	6–8
Hemopathology: 1+ leptocytosis and anisocytosis.		

Biochemical Profile		Reference Range
Gluc (mg/dl)	88	65–122
BUN (mg/dl)	17	7–28
Creat (mg/dl)	1.1	0.9–1.7
Ca (mg/dl)	10.2	9.0–11.2
Phos (mg/dl)	3.5	2.8–6.1
TP (g/dl)	**4.1**	5.4–7.4
Alb (g/dl)	**2.3**	2.7–4.5
Glob (g/dl)	**1.8**	1.9–3.4
T. Bili (mg/dl)	0.3	0–0.4
Chol (mg/dl)	188	130–370
ALT (IU/L)	35	10–120
ALP (IU/L)	40	35–280
Na (mEq/L)	**144**	145–158
K (mEq/L)	**4.0**	4.1–5.5
CL (mEq/L)	107	106–127
TCO₂ (mEq/L)	18	14–27

Coagulation Data		Reference Range
Activated clotting time (sec)	**>180**	72–86
PT (seconds)	**>180**	6.4–7.4
aPTT (seconds)	**>180**	9–11
Fibrinogen (mg/dl)	300	100–400
Bleeding Time (minutes)	4	1–5

Interpretive Discussion

Hematology

The anemia is nonregenerative as the erythrocyte indices are normal and the reticulocyte count is normal. Mild neutrophilia, monocytosis, and lymphopenia are indicative of a stress leukogram. The plasma and serum protein are low, with equal deficiency of globulin and albumin, suggesting blood loss as the cause of anemia. The anemia is likely too acute for there to be a regenerative response. Aspiration of the subcutaneous mass confirmed the presence of blood.

Biochemical Profile

The protein changes discussed above indicate subacute blood loss, with fluid shifting and dilution of plasma protein resulting in anemia and hypoproteinemia. The mild decrease in sodium and potassium are insignificant.

Coagulation Data

The coagulation data indicates either a deficiency of multiple coagulation factors, or a single factor deficiency of the common pathway. Platelets are normal in number, and, no large forms are seen in peripheral blood. Bleeding time is normal and in the face of normal platelet concentration, indicates that platelet function is also normal. The most common cause of a severe coagulopathy with normal platelets and normal hepatic enzyme activities is vitamin K antagonism.

Summary

This dog was exposed to diphacinone, a rodentocide that is a vitamin K antagonist; coagulation times returned to normal following administration of vitamin K.

CASE 14

Signalment: 2-month-old female horse
History: Off feed
Physical Examination: Depressed, evidence of diarrhea

Hematology		Reference Range
PCV (%)	14	32–52
Hgb (g/dl)	6.5	11–19
NCC (×10³/μl)	6.5	5.5–12.5
Segs (×10³/μl)	4.7	2.7–6.7
Monos (×10³/μl)	0.1	0–0.8
Lymphs (×10³/μl)	1.6	1.5–5.5
NRBCs (×10³/μl)	0.1	0
Platelets (×10³/μl)	14	100–600
TP (P) (g/dl)	6.3	6–8

Hemopathology: mod toxic neutrophils, few reactive lymphs, mod Howell-Jolly bodies, few echinocytes, marked anisocytosis.

Biochemical Profile		Reference Range
Gluc (mg/dl)	91	70–110
BUN (mg/dl)	40	14–27
Creat (mg/dl)	2.1	1.1–2.0
Ca (mg/dl)	9.7	11.0–13.7
Phos (mg/dl)	6.3	1.9–4.1
TP (g/dl)	4.6	5.8–7.6
Alb (g/dl)	2.2	2.7–3.7
Glob (g/dl)	2.4	2.6–4.6
T. Bili (mg/dl)	3.2	0.6–2.1
AST (IU/L)	280	185–300
GGT (IU/L)	28	7–17
SDH (IU/L)	27	0–9
CK (IU/L)	169	130–470
Na (mEq/L)	120	133–145
K (mEq/L)	3.8	2.2–4.6
CL (mEq/L)	84	100–111
TCO₂ (mEq/L)	11.0	24–34
An. gap	28.8	5–15
Calc. Osmolality (mOsm/kg)	250	280–310
Amylase (IU/L)	34	0–87
Lipase (IU/L)	534	ND*
Grossly lipemic serum		

*ND - Not determined for foals.

Blood Gas Data (arterial)		Reference Range
pH	7.282	7.38–7.46
pCO₂ (mmHg)	20.6	35–47
pO₂ (mmHg)	60.9	67–96
HCO₃ (mEq/L)	9.3	22–30

Coagulation Profile		Reference Range
PT (seconds)	14.6	9.5–11.5
aPTT (seconds)	39.8	24–45
Fibrinogen (mg/dl)	500	100–400
FDPs (μg/ml)	>10 & <40	ND*

* ND - Not determined for foals.

Abdominal Fluid Analysis	
Color	**Red**
Clarity	**Opaque**
NCC (/μl)	**16,000**
TP (g/dl)	**5.7**
PCV	**13%**

Comments: Erythrophagia and platelets noted in film.

Interpretive Discussion

Hematology

There is a marked anemia. While it is not unusual for neonatal animals to have a "congenital anemia" due to iron deficiency, the PCV is much lower than is typically encountered by this physiological change. The presence of anisocytosis leads one to suspect that there may be a regenerative response, for which evaluation of the MCV would be useful. The presence of nucleated erythrocytes in the peripheral blood is uncommon in horses, but occasionally seen in foals with profound regenerative responses, or with damage to the bone marrow endothelium, as might occur with sepsis. Combined decreases in PCV and serum proteins may indicate hemorrhage. There is a marked thrombocytopenia, which may be due to decreased production or increased consumption; thrombocytopenia is severe enough to be resulting in blood loss. Refer to the discussion of the coagulation profile for more on this matter.

Biochemical Profile

The BUN and serum creatinine concentrations are increased, but the nature of this azotemia cannot be definitively differentiated without a urinalysis.

There is hypocalcemia and hyperphosphatemia. This combination of mineral abnormalities may be seen in nutritional secondary hyperparathyroidism due to excessive dietary phosphorus. However, higher serum phosphorus concentrations are commonly observed in growing animals, and hypocalcemia may also be due to uptake by widespread damaged tissues, decreased intake with anorexia, or to an apparent decrease due to hypoalbuminemia.

Serum total protein concentration is decreased, including both hypoalbuminemia and hypoglobulinemia. Low serum albumin may be hepatocellular dysfunction or cachexia and decreased albumin synthesis. Alternatively, there may be pathologic albumin loss due to gastrointestinal or renal disease. Low serum globulin in a 2-month-old foal is not due to failure of passive transfer, but may be due to decreased production, malnutrition, or pathologic loss. Loss of all proteins would be expected with hemorrhage, which could also account for the profound anemia. This is the most likely cause.

The serum total bilirubin concentration is increased, with only a mild increase in serum GGT activity. This may reflect hyperbilirubinemia of fasting in an anorexic patient. However, SDH activity is increased, indicating hepatocellular damage.

Serum sodium and chloride concentrations are decreased. This is commonly observed in young animals with an enterotoxigenic or secretory diarrhea. This may also be due to gastrointestinal stasis, a third space accumulation in the abdominal cavity, as well as to decreased intake. One would typically expect a hyperkalemia to occur in secretory diarrhea, owing to acidosis-induced intercompartmental exchange. Hypokalemia may be expected in third space syndromes, owing to potassium loss and renal decompensation. It is possible to observe normokalemia with concomitant potassium loss and metabolic acidosis, wherein redistribution of potassium from the intracellular to the extracellular fluid compartment obscures the whole body potassium deficit. There is evidence in support of abdominal hemorrhage and third spacing due either to acute pancreatitis or a gastric ulcer (see below).

Marked lipemia is often seen in ponies with starvation and metabolic disease, but is unusual in horses. In other species, hyperlipidemia may occur due to impaired triglyceride clearance associated with endotoxemia. One should consider other potential causes of hyperlipidemia such as pancreatitis. In this case, serum amylase activity is normal, but lipase activity may be increased. There is evidence of recent hemorrhage into the abdominal cavity, which could be related to acute pancreatitis, but is more often due, in diseased foals, to a bleeding gastric ulcer. The low calculated osmolality would be expected, given the hyponatremia and hypochloremia.

Blood Gas Data

There is an increased anion gap metabolic acidosis with respiratory compensation. This is consistent with a secretory diarrhea, complicated by hypovolemia and/or sepsis. If there were gastrointestinal stasis, one might expect an alkalosis. If there were a ruptured urinary bladder, one might expect a metabolic acidosis with hyperkalemia. The increased anion gap may result from sepsis, with hypovolemia and lactic acidosis due to reduced tissue perfusion and/or the metabolic effects of endotoxemia. The decreased oxygen tension may indicate respiratory compromise as well, or inadequate oxygenation with assisted ventilation.

Coagulation Data

The prothrombin time is prolonged slightly, the activated partial thromboplastin time is normal, and the FDP concentration is in an intermediate range. These findings may indicate disseminated intravascular coagulation, particularly in light of the severe thrombocytopenia, wherein Factor VII levels are becoming depleted, thereby prolonging the PT, but other coagulation factor concentrations are adequate to maintain a normal APTT. The concurrent observation of thrombocytopenia and findings consistent with blood loss anemia support a diagnosis of DIC with pathologic hemorrhage.

Summary

Enterotoxigenic *E. coli* diarrhea, pancreatitis, hepatitis, and DIC were findings confirmed at necropsy. On necropsy, the pancreas was 5 to 6 times normal size and the liver was swollen. Histopathology showed necrosis and inflammation of the pancreas, diffuse mesenteric steatitis, fat necrosis and fat saponification, inflammation of the liver with thrombi in central veins and associated focal ischemic necrosis.

CASE 15

Signalment: 3-year-old spayed female cocker spaniel
History: Left in owner's car in shopping mall parking lot for approximately 3 hours on a hot summer afternoon.
Physical Examination: Depressed and mildly dehydrated

Hematology		Reference Range
PCV (%)	**58**	37–55
NCC (×10³/μl)	16.0	6–17
Segs (×10³/μl)	**13.4**	3–11.5
Monos (×10³/μl)	**1.6**	0.1–1.3
Lymphs (×10³/μl)	1.0	1–4.8
Platelets (×10³/μl)	Adequate	200–500

Biochemical Profile		Reference Range
Gluc (mg/dl)	**142**	65–122
BUN (mg/dl)	**62**	7–28
Creat (mg/dl)	**3.0**	0.9–1.7
Ca (mg/dl)	**8.4**	9.0–11.2
Phos (mg/dl)	4.9	2.8–6.1
TP (g/dl)	**9.4**	5.4–7.4
Alb (g/dl)	**5.4**	2.7–4.5
Glob (g/dl)	**4.0**	1.9–3.4
T. Bili (mg/dl)	0.4	0–0.4
Chol (mg/dl)	160	130–370
ALT (IU/L)	**178**	10–120
ALP (IU/L)	60	35–280
Na (mEq/L)	**164**	145–158
K (mEq/L)	5.4	4.1–5.5
CL (mEq/L)	124	106–127
TCO₂ (mEq/L)	14	14–27
An. gap (mEq/L)	**31.4**	8–25
Meas. Osmolality (mOsm/kg)	**358**	290–310
Calc. Osmolality (mOsm/kg)	**344**	290–310
Osmole gap (mOsm/kg)	**14**	0–10

Blood Gas Data (arterial)		Reference Range
pH	**7.09**	7.33–7.45
PCO₂ (mmHg)	**46**	24–39
HCO₃ (mEq/L)	**13**	14–24

Urinalysis				
Color	Dk yellow	**Urine Sediment**		
		WBCs/hpf	2–3	
Transparency	Cloudy	RBCs/hpf	4–5	
Sp. Gr.	1.011	Epith cells/hpf	2–3	
Protein	1+	Casts/lpf	**2–3 fine granular**	
Gluc	Neg			
Bilirubin	Neg	Crystals	2+ Ca oxalate	
Blood	Neg	Bacteria	0	
pH	5.5			

Interpretive Discussion

Hematology

Hemoconcentration is indicated by the increased PCV and physical signs of dehydration. Mild neutrophilia, monocytosis, and borderline lymphopenia is probably secondary to stress or increased endogenous or exogenous corticosteroids.

Biochemical Profile

There is a mild hyperglycemia, which may be due to a catecholaminergic or steroid stress response.

The BUN and serum creatinine concentrations are increased. See discussion of urinalysis below to explain whether the azotemia is likely prerenal, renal, or postrenal.

Hyperalbuminemia indicates dehydration. In this case, hyperglobulememia is also likely caused by dehydration.

There is a mild hypocalcemia in the face of hyperalbuminemia due to dehydration. Thus, serum calcium concentration is truly decreased. This is often seen in heat-stressed animals, subsequent to widespread tissue damage and precipitation of calcium salts in ischemic areas.

The small increase in serum ALT activity may not be significant, or may reflect some hepatocellular damage.

The hypernatremia, in concert with other signs of dehydration, indicates a hypertonic dehydration. This is commonly seen in heat-stressed dogs owing to increased insensible losses of water, in excess of solute, due to hyperventilatory evaporation.

The measured and calculated osmolality values are increased, consistent with hypertonic dehydration. However, the osmole gap is also increased, indicating the accumulation of unmeasured osmotically active solutes in the blood. The anion gap is likewise increased, and given the dehydration and probable tissue hypoperfusion, some degree of lactic acidosis is likely.

Blood Gas Data

There is a combined metabolic (decreased bicarbonate) and respiratory (increased pCO_2) acidosis. The metabolic acidosis results from lactic acidosis due to tissue hypoperfusion. The respiratory acidosis suggests compromised pulmonary function.

Urinalysis

The presence of 1+ proteinuria with a specific gravity of 1.011 indicates significant urinary protein loss. The fine granular casts indicate tubular epithelial damage. The isosthenuric specific gravity in the face of dehydration and azotemia, yet in the absence of electrolyte depletion, suggests renal disease as well. This is likely a case of acute renal failure secondary to heat stress. The presence of calcium oxalate crystals may have no importance, or may represent one potential route of calcium loss due to renal tubular damage associated with the hypocalcemia.

Summary

Heat stress, hypertonic dehydration, and acute renal failure. If one did not have the history given, or doubted its veracity, laboratory findings like these would strongly suggest antifreeze intoxication. One could analyze serum for ethylene glycol concentration to definitively rule this possibility in or out.

CASE 16

Signalment: 4-year-old intact male dog
History: Experiencing intermittent periods of weakness and lameness
Physical Examination: Mild dehydration, foul smelling breath, teeth covered with tartar

Hematology		Reference Range
PCV (%)	11	37–55
Hgb (g/dl)	**4.0**	12–18
RBC (×10⁶/μl)	**1.64**	5.5–8.5
MCV (fl)	67	60–72
MCHC (g/dl)	36	34–38
Retics (/μl)	**13.1**	< 60
NCC (×10³/μl)	8.7	6–17
Segs (×10³/μl)	7.7	3–11.5
Bands (×10³/μl)	0.1	0–0.3
Monos (×10³/μl)	0.3	0.1–1.3
Lymphs (×10³/μl)	**0.4**	1–4.8
Eos (×10³/μl)	0.2	0.1–1.2
Platelets (×10³/μl)	370	200–500
TP (P) (g/dl)	6.8	6–8

Hemopathology: Slight anisocytosis and slight polychromasia

Biochemical Profile		Reference Range
Gluc (mg/dl)	91	65–122
BUN (mg/dl)	**183 (65.3)**	7–28 (2.5–10.0 mmol/L)
Creat (mg/dl)	**8.1 (716)**	0.9–1.7 (79–150 μmol/L)
Ca (mg/dl)	**8.2 (2.05)**	9.0–11.2 (2.25–2.8 mmol/L)
Phos (mg/dl)	**17.2 (5.5)**	2.8–6.1 (0.9–2.9 mmol/L)
TP (g/dl)	5.8	5.4–7.4
Alb (g/dl)	3.2	2.7–4.5
Glob (g/dl)	2.6	1.9–3.4
T. Bili (mg/dl)	0.4	0–0.4
Chol (mg/dl)	180	130–370
ALT (IU/L)	19	10–120
AST (IU/L)	17	16–40
ALP (IU/L)	40	35–280
Na (mEq/L)	146	145–158
K (mEq/L)	5.0	4.1–5.5
CL (mEq/L)	115	106–127
TCO₂ (mEq/L)	16	14–27
An. gap (mEq/L)	20	8–25

Urinalysis (catheterized)			
Color	Yellow	**Urine Sediment**	
Transparency	Clear	WBCs/hpf	3–5
Sp. Gr.	**1.008**	RBCs/hpf	2–3
Protein	Trace	Epith cells/hpf	0
Gluc	Negative	Casts/lpf	0
Bilirubin	Negative	Crystals	0
Blood	Negative	Bacteria	0
pH	5.0		

Interpretive Discussion

Hematology

The nonregenerative anemia is secondary to chronic renal disease. Decreased erythropoietin production by the kidneys is a major factor leading to anemia in animals with chronic renal disease. The severity of anemia is unusual for chronic renal disease. Such anemias are typically of mild to moderate severity. Other causes of nonregenerative anemia should also be considered in this case.

The cause of the lymphopenia is increased blood steroid concentration associated with stress. The leukocyte response in not a typical steroid-mediated response in that a mature neutrophilia typically accompanies lymphopenia. It is likely that the animal's resting neutrophil concentration was low normal and it has approximately doubled due to the steroid influence.

Biochemical Profile

The triad of BUN, creatinine, and phosphorus concentrations is markedly increased indicating decreased glomerular filtration. These products are passively filtered by the glomerulus, and any cause of decreased glomerular filtration will result in retention of these analytes in the blood. In light of the urine specific gravity in the isosthenuric range, primary renal azotemia is most likely.

At least two mechanisms have played a role in causing the hypocalcemia. The phosphorus concentration is markedly increased, and the Ca × P product is 141. When this product exceeds 70, calcium and phosphorus precipitate in soft tissues, decreasing the serum calcium concentration. In addition, chronic renal disease may result in decreased activation of vitamin D by the kidneys (i.e., conversion of 25-hydroxycholecalciferol to 1,25-dihydroxycholecalciferol). Decreased activated vitamin D results in decreased absorption of calcium from the intestinal tract.

Urinalysis

A urine specific gravity in the isosthenuric range in an azotemic animal suggests an inability to concentrate urine. Animals with prerenal azotemia due to decreased renal perfusion (e.g., dehydration, cardiac insufficiency, circulatory shock) should be conserving water and concentrating urine. The urine specific gravity is a key to properly interpreting the cause of the azotemia in this case.

Urine sediment–Small numbers of leukocytes and erythrocytes are normal in urine. These numbers must be interpreted in light of the urine concentration and the technique used to concentrate the sediment. Leukocyte numbers may be slightly increased in this case, suggesting inflammation in the urinary tract.

Summary

These data suggest chronic renal failure. Chronicity is suggested by the nonregenerative anemia, which would not be present with acute renal failure. Postmortem diagnosis in this case was chronic interstitial nephritis. No lesions suggesting suppurative inflammation in the urinary tract were found.

CASE 17

Signalment: 9-year-old intact female dog
History: Abscess on rear leg 2 months ago. Intermittent vomiting began 2 days ago.
Physical Examination: Popliteal and cervical lymph nodes are enlarged.

Hematology		Reference Range
PCV (%)	**35**	37–55
Hgb (g/dl)	12.1	12–18
RBC (×10⁶/µl)	5.6	5.5–8.5
MCV (fl)	62	60–72
MCHC (g/dl)	36	34–38
Retics (/µl)	22.4	< 60
NCC (×10³/µl)	13	6–17
Segs (×10³/µl)	9.4	3–11.5
Bands (×10³/µl)	0.1	0–0.3
Monos (×10³/µl)	0.8	0.1–1.3
Lymphs (×10³/µl)	2.4	1–4.8
Eos (×10³/µl)	0.3	0.1–1.2
Platelets (×10³/µl)	250	200–500
TP (P) (g/dl)	6.2	6–8
Hemopathology: Normal		

Biochemical Profile		Reference Range
Gluc (mg/dl)	89	65–122
BUN (mg/dl)	**114 (40.7)**	7–28 (2.5–10.0 mmol/L)
Creat (mg/dl)	**3.2 (283)**	0.9–1.7 (79–150 µmol/L)
Ca (mg/dl)	**8.5 (2.12)**	9.0–11.2 (2.25–2.8 mmol/L)
Phos (mg/dl)	**8.8 (2.84)**	2.8–6.1 (0.9–2.9 mmol/L)
TP (g/dl)	5.2	5.4–7.4
Alb (g/dl)	**1.2**	2.7–4.5
Glob (g/dl)	**4.0**	1.9–3.4
T. Bili (mg/dl)	0.3	0–0.4
Chol (mg/dl)	**582 (15.1)**	130–370 (3.4–9.6 mmol/L)
ALT (IU/L)	18	10–120
AST (IU/L)	20	16–40
ALP (IU/L)	22	35–280
Na (mEq/L)	**142**	145–158
K (mEq/L)	4.7	4.1–5.5
CL (mEq/L)	120	106–127
TCO₂ (mEq/L)	18	14–27
An. gap (mEq/L)	9	8–25
Amylase (IU/L)	**1530**	50–1250
Lipase (IU/L)	**720**	30–560

Urinalysis (catheterized)			
Color	Yellow	**Urine Sediment**	
Transparency	Cloudy	WBCs/hpf	0
Sp. Gr.	**1.021**	RBCs/hpf	0
Protein	**4+**	Epith cells/hpf	0
Gluc	Negative	Casts/lpf	2–3 granular
Bilirubin	Negative	Crystals	0
Blood	Negative	Bacteria	0
pH	6.0		
protein/ creatinine ratio	5.4		

Interpretive Discussion

Hematology

A mild nonregenerative anemia (reticulocyte count is in the normal range) is present. This should prompt an evaluation for endocrine disease, renal disease, and chronic inflammatory disease as potential causes. In this case, chronic renal disease is probably the underlying cause. There is no evidence of current inflammatory disease in the leukogram.

Biochemical Profile

This azotemia indicated by increased concentrations of BUN, and creatinine should be classified as renal since urine concentration is not adequate (i.e., <1.030), suggesting a loss of renal concentrating ability.

The hypocalcemia is probably due to two factors. The calcium X phosphorus product is 75. When this product exceeds 70, precipitation of calcium and phosphorus in soft tissues can occur, and decreased serum calcium concentrations may result. In addition, activation of vitamin D by the kidney is decreased in chronic renal disease, resulting in decreased absorption of calcium from the small intestine.

The hyperphosphatemia is due to decreased glomerular filtration rate (GFR). In this case, glomerular disease has caused decreased GFR and subsequent hyperphosphatemia.

In light of the marked proteinuria, the most likely cause of the hypoproteinemia and hypoalbuminemia is renal protein loss, most likely due to glomerular disease. The hyperglobulinemia most likely resulted from chronic antigenic stimulation. History of a previous abscess and subsequent lymph node enlargement are compatible with such antigenic stimulation (i.e., the original infection may not have been completely eliminated, resulting in chronic antigenic stimulation and hyperplasia in lymphoid tissue). Such chronic antigenic stimulation can predispose to some forms of glomerular disease.

Hypercholesterolemia is probably a component of nephrotic syndrome. Nephrotic syndrome, a group of abnormalities that may be associated with serious glomerular disease, includes hypoalbuminemia, proteinuria, hypercholesterolemia and edema. In this case, edema was not observed; however, presence of the other three components is still suggestive of this syndrome. Edema is not likely to occur until the albumin is below 1.0 g/dl. The mechanism causing hypercholesterolemia in this syndrome has not been identified.

The cause of mild hyponatremia is not certain in this case. Renal Na loss is a possible cause. If edema were present, it is possible that dilution of extracellular Na in this fluid (third-spacing) could result in decreased serum Na concentration. Edema was, however, not evident in this case, and, even in animals with edema, hyponatremia is not common.

Serum amylase and lipase activities are commonly increased in animals with decreased GFR. Although other causes of increased activities such as pancreatitis could be considered in this case, the clinical presentation and other laboratory data are more compatible with decreased GFR resulting in increased amylase and lipase activities.

Urinalysis

Urine concentrating ability is inadequate. If the azotemia in this dog were due to prerenal causes such as dehydration, cardiac insufficiency, or circulatory shock, urine specific gravity should be >1.030. The specific gravity suggests inadequate concentrating ability and renal azotemia. Post-renal azotemia is ruled out by the demonstration of a patent urethra via catheterization and by the absence of evidence of urine leakage into tissues or the abdomen. Lack of concentrating ability results from loss of nephrons and/or tubular damage. Both of these alterations are probably occurring in this dog. Although the disease is primarily glomerular, severe damage to glomeruli results in secondary tubular damage and in loss of nephrons.

A 4+ protein in a moderately dilute urine and a urine protein/creatinine ratio (UPC) of 5.4 are evidence of severe proteinuria. In the absence of evidence of hemorrhage or inflammation (i.e., increased erythrocyte or leukocyte numbers in the urine sediment), a UPC >1.0 is abnormal in the dog, and a UPC >5.0 is suggestive of glomerular disease. A UPC of >15 is diagnostic for glomerular disease.

Summary

Renal biopsy revealed amyloidosis. Chronic infection resulting in chronic antigenic stimulation probably predisposed the dog to this disease. The lymph node enlargement was most likely due to hyperplasia secondary to chronic antigenic stimulation. The combination of hypoalbuminemia, proteinuria, and hypercholesterolemia suggest imminent onset of nephrotic syndrome.

CASE 18

Signalment: 13-year-old castrated male cat
History: Rear leg paralysis. Dyspnea. Vomiting.

Physical Examination: Lethargy and dyspnea. Systolic murmur detected.

Hematology	Day 1		Reference Range
PCV (%)	35		24–45
Hgb (g/dl)	11.3		8–15
RBC (×10⁶/µl)	8.05		5–11
MCV (fl)	44		39–50
MCHC (g/dl)	32		33–37
NCC (×10³/µl)	18.1		5.5–19.5
Segs (×10³/µl)	**16.3**		2.5–12.5
Monos (×10³/µl)	0.5		0–0.8
Lymphs (×10³/µl)	**0.9**		1.5–7.0
Basiphils (×10³/µl)	0.2		Rare
NRBC (×10³/µl)	**0.2**		0
Platelets (×10³/µl)	Adequate		
TP (P) (g/dl)	7.2		6–8
Hemopathology: Normal			

Biochemical Profile	Day 1	Day 3	Reference Range
Gluc (mg/dl)	**153 (8.4)**	**360 (19.8)**	67–124 (3.7–6.8 mmol/L)
BUN (mg/dl)	**46 (16.4)**	**137 (48.9)**	17–32 (6.1–11.4 mmol/L)
Creat (mg/dl)	**2.9 (256)**	**9.8 (866)**	0.9–2.1 (80–186 µmol/L)
Ca (mg/dl)	**8.4 (2.12)**	**4.9 (1.22)**	8.5–11 (2.12–2.75 mmol/L)
Phos (mg/dl)	**8.0 (2.6)**	**16.1 (5.2)**	3.3–7.8 (1.1–2.5 mmol/L)
TP (g/dl)	6.9	**5.4**	5.9–8.1
Alb (g/dl)	2.8	2.4	2.3–3.9
Glob (g/dl)	4.1	3.0	2.9–4.4
T. Bili (mg/dl)	0.2	0.3	0–0.3
Chol (mg/dl)	192	151	60–220
ALT (IU/L)	**158**	**294**	30–100
AST (IU/L)	**461**	**643**	14–38
ALP (IU/L)	54	25	6–106
GGT (IU/L)	0	1	0–1
CK (IU/L)	**45,313**	**350,930**	60–300
Na (mEq/L)	150	139	146–160
K (mEq/L)	4.9	**6.6**	3.7–5.4
CL (mEq/L)	119	**99**	112–129
TCO₂ (mEq/L)	19.2	15.9	14–23
An. gap (mEq/L)	17	**31**	10–27

Urinalysis (cystocentesis)	Day 1	Day 3	Urine Sediment	Day 1	Day 3
Color	Dark yellow	Light yellow	WBCs/hpf	15–20	0–1
Transparency	Hazy	Clear	RBCs/hpf	35–50	5–10
Sp. Gr.	1.050	1.010	Epith cells/hpf	0	0
Protein	2+	1+	Casts/lpf	Few granular	0
Gluc	4+	4+	Crystals	0	0
Bilirubin	Negative	Negative	Bacteria	0	0
Blood	4+	4+	Ketones		
PH	5.5	5.0			

Fractional excretion	Day 1		Reference Range
Na (%)	7.2		<1.0
K (%)	165.1		5–20
P (%)	68.6		<7–21
Ca (%)	10.5		<1.0

Coagulation Data	Day 1	Day 3	Reference Range
PT (seconds)	10.0	8.9	7–11.5
aPTT (seconds)	8.2	16.5	10–15

Endocrine Data	Day 1	Day 3	Reference Range
Total T4 (µg/dl)		1.34	1.2–4.8

Interpretive Discussion

Hematology

In light of normal values for other erythrocyte measurements, the slightly decreased MCHC is probably not significant. Mature neutrophilia and lymphopenia are typical of a stress leukogram. The basophils are probably not significant. Occasionally, nucleated RBCs may be found in the blood of normal animals. In the absence of anemia or other erythrocyte abnormalities, the nucleated RBCs noted in this cat are not important.

Biochemical Profile

The cat is hyperglycemic on Days 1 and 3. This abnormality could be due to severe excitement or stress with resulting increased epinephrine or corticosteroid levels, respectively. The leukogram is suggestive of stress. The presence of ketonuria on Day 1 suggests that diabetes mellitus should also be considered. Although this cat's blood glucose concentration on Day 1 is not above the renal threshold, detection of glucosuria on this day suggests that the cat may have had periods with higher blood glucose concentrations or that this cat has an abnormally low renal threshold for glucose.

The cat has an azotemia which progresses from mild to severe. Since urine specific gravity is high on Day 1, the azotemia on that day appears to be prerenal. Urine specific gravity is in the isosthenuric range on Day 3 and may be of renal origin; however, the cat had received fluid therapy, and this, rather than renal failure, may have caused the low urine specific gravity on this day.

Hypocalcemia progresses from mild on Day 1 to marked on Day 3. While ethylene glycol toxicosis may result in hypocalcemia and causes severe azotemia, rear leg paralysis and increased CK activity are not associated with ethylene glycol toxicosis. The Ca X P product on Day 1 is 67 on Day 1 and 79 by Day 3. Precipitation of Ca and P in the tissues may, therefore, be occurring on Day 3 and may, in part, explain the decreasing Ca concentration. Massive tissue destruction, as evidenced by increased CK activity, may have resulted in calcium precipitation in damaged tissues and subsequent hypocalcemia.

Hyperphosphatemia resulted from decreased glomerular filtration rate. Maintenance of normal serum P concentration depends on normal glomerular clearance of P.

Total serum protein concentration was normal on Day 1 but decreased by Day 3. Although both albumin and globulin concentrations remained within reference ranges, concentrations of both of these proteins decreased due to fluid therapy and subsequent expansion of blood volume. In light of normal serum albumin and globulin concentrations, the significance of the hypoproteinemia is questionable.

Increased serum ALT activity suggests mild hepatocyte injury that progressed to moderate.

The combination of increased serum AST and CK activities indicates muscle injury. Since CK has a short half-life (less than four hours), the extremely high CK activity implies active muscle damage. AST is also present in hepatocytes, and hepatic injury is an alternate explanation for the increased serum AST activity, but, in light of the increased serum CK activity, muscle origin is most likely.

Hyponatremia on Day 3 may be due to renal loss (see fractional excretion results). Since hypochloremia is also evident, vomiting could also be a cause of Na loss. Hypochloremia on Day 3 may be due to both renal loss and vomiting.

Hyperkalemia on Day 3 may be due to several different causes. Since the cat is in renal failure, kidneys may not be excreting K normally. This cat also had a significant degree of tissue necrosis that could have resulted in release of K from dead or dying cells.

The increased anion gap suggests increased concentrations of anions such as ketones, uremic acids, phosphate, sulfate, or lactate. Ketones are not present in the urine of this cat on Day 3, and a significant ketosis is, therefore, not likely. Since the cat is severely azotemic, concentrations of uremic acids are probably increased. Serum phosphorus concentration confirms that increased phosphate is contributing to the anion gap. The final diagnosis suggested that this cat had significant tissue damage, and this probably increased serum sulfate concentrations. Hypoxia was also a component of this cat's disease; therefore, lactic acidosis was also occurring.

Urinalysis

The implications of the urine specific gravities were discussed in the interpretation of this cat's azotemia. The cat has proteinuria and hematuria on both days and pyuria on Day 1. These abnormalities suggest urinary tract inflammation. Cystitis or pyelonephritis are possible causes of

this inflammation. The protein concentration decreased between Days 1 and 3, but this probably reflects the change in the concentration of the urine with more dilution of protein on Day 3. Both pyuria and hematuria probably contributed to the proteinuria. Other causes of proteinuria such as glomerular or tubular disease cannot be eliminated. The dipstick test for blood was equally increased on Days 1 and 3, but the RBC concentration decreased markedly between these days. This suggests that the positive test is due to either hemoglobinuria or myoglobinuria. In light of the apparent muscle injury (increased CK), myoglobinuria is most likely.

Glucosuria is marked on both days. On Day 3, this reflects a blood glucose concentration which exceeds the renal threshold. The glucosuria is more difficult to explain on Day 1, when the blood glucose is below the renal threshold. While it is possible that this cat has a lowered renal threshold, it is also possible blood glucose concentrations were fluctuating on Day 1 with periods above the renal threshold occurring.

Presence of a few granular cast suggests tubular damage.

The significance of the positive urine ketone reaction is considered in the discussion of hyperglycemia.

Fractional excretions of Na, K, P, and Ca are increased. This indicates abnormal reabsorption of these electrolytes and, in this case, is probably due to acute renal damage.

Coagulation Data

The activated partial thromboplastin time (APTT) is slightly decreased on Day 1 and probably reflects this cat's hypercoagulable condition. The mechanism of this change is not known but may be related to this cat's cardiac problem (see Summary and Outcome). This cat was treated with streptokinase between Days 1 and 3, and this treatment increases APTT and PT, and return of APTT to within the reference range on Day 3 may have resulted from this treatment; however, the absence of a longer PT on Day 1 as compared to Day 3 makes a significant effect of streptokinase treatment less certain.

Summary

Clinical diagnosis was restrictive cardiomyopathy with aortic thromboemboli (saddle and renal thrombosis and pulmonary thromboembolism). Restrictive cardiomyopathy predisposes to thrombosis. In this case, the thrombotic disease involved the kidneys and resulted in acute renal failure. In addition, hypoxia occurred in other tissues including the muscles of the rear legs. This resulted in increased serum activities of AST and CK. Necropsy examination was not performed.

CASE 19

Signalment: 11-year-old FS canine
History: Weight loss and polyuria
Physical Examination: Thin, slightly dehydrated

Hematology		Reference Range
PCV (%)	36.0	37–55
Hgb (g/dl)	12.5	12–18
RBC (×10⁶/μl)	5.38	5.5–8.5
MCV (fl)	67.0	60–72
MCHC (g/dl)	35.0	34–38
NCC (×10³/μl)	7.0	6–17
Segs (×10³/μl)	6.1	3–11.5
Bands (×10³/μl)	0.1	0–0.3
Monos (×10³/μl)	0.2	0.1–1.3
Lymphs (×10³/μl)	**0.5**	1–4.8
Eos (×10³/μl)	0.1	0.1–1.2
Platelets (×10³/μl)	400	200–500
TP (P) (g/dl)	8.1	6–8

Biochemical Profile		Reference Range
Gluc (mg/dl)	112	65–122
BUN (mg/dl)	**216 (77.1)**	7–28 (2.5–10.0 mmol/L)
Creat (mg/dl)	**15.6 (1379)**	0.9–1.7 (79–150 μmol/L)
Ca (mg/dl)	**12.1 (3.0)**	9.0–11.2 (2.25–2.8 mmol/L)
Phos (mg/dl)	**20.9 (6.75)**	2.8–6.1 (0.9–2.9 mmol/L)
TP (g/dl)	6.9	5.4–7.4
Alb (g/dl)	4.0	2.7–4.5
Glob (g/dl)	2.9	1.9–3.4
T. Bili (mg/dl)	0.4	0–0.4
Chol (mg/dl)	335	130–370
ALT (IU/L)	73	10–120
AST (IU/L)	25	16–40
ALP (IU/L)	**662**	35–280
GGT (IU/L)	**8**	0–6
Na (mEq/L)	**144**	145–158
K (mEq/L)	**6.2**	4.1–5.5
CL (mEq/L)	**98**	106–127
TCO₂ (mEq/L)	**13.1**	14–27
An. gap (mEq/L)	**39**	8–25
Amylase (IU/L)	866	50–1250
Lipase (IU/L)	386	30–560

Urinalysis			
Color	Yellow	**Urine Sediment**	
Transparency	Cloudy	WBCs/hpf	1–2
Sp. Gr.	**1.011**	RBCs/hpf	1–2
Protein	**3+**	Epith cells/hpf	5–8
Gluc	Negative	Casts/lpf	**0–1 coarse granular and waxy**
Bilirubin	1+	Crystals	Negative
Blood	Trace	Bacteria	Negative
pH	6.0		
UPC	**11.1**		

Interpretive Discussion

Hematology

The PCV is marginally decreased, but without a reticulocyte count it is difficult to classify the regenerative response. A marginal normocytic, normochromic anemia is observed in renal failure, for which there are other indications in the laboratory data.

The lymphopenia indicates a steroid response.

Biochemical Profile

The serum glucose concentration is normal.

The BUN, serum creatinine, and serum phosphorus values are markedly increased. These findings are consistent with decreased glomerular filtration rate. However, one cannot differentiate the nature of the azotemia (prerenal, renal, or postrenal) based on these findings alone. Refer to the discussion of urinalysis results for further interpretation.

Serum total calcium is mildly increased, for which one should consider hypercalcemia of malignancy, hypoadrenocorticism, renal failure, vitamin D toxicosis, or primary hyperparathyroidism.

Serum cholesterol concentration is increased, and total bilirubin is at the upper end of the reference range. Together with a significant increase in serum ALP activity and mild increase in GGT activity, this is consistent with cholestasis. However, because AST and ALT activities are normal, there is not likely any hepatocellular damage. ALP and GGT activities may also be increased by corticosteroids.

Serum Na and Cl are decreased in concentration, while serum K is increased. The Na:K ratio is 23.2, which may indicate hypoadrenocorticism. Alternatively, renal disease may result in a functional hypoadrenocorticism due to inability of the damaged renal tubules to respond appropriately to mineralocorticoids or may be due to a simple loss of sodium and retention of potassium because of renal disease and oliguria. The serum total CO_2 is decreased, indicating a metabolic acidosis, while the anion gap is increased, indicating the accumulation of organic anions. Acidosis may result in hyperkalemia as well.

The serum calculated osmolality is increased, predominantly because of the profound azotemia. Likewise, the increased anion gap is due to retention of urinary metabolic products.

Serum amylase and lipase activities are normal, and while not definitive, lessen the probability for pancreatitis.

Urinalysis

The urinary specific gravity is in the isosthenuric range, and there is 3+ proteinuria in the absence of significant hematuria or pyuria. The urinary protein:creatinine ratio is 11.1, which is significantly increased. The mild bilirubinuria is likely significant considering the low specific gravity. The coarse granular and waxy casts also definitively indicate renal tubular damage. Together with the marked azotemia, these findings support a diagnosis of renal disease.

Summary

Malignant fibrous histiocytoma of both kidneys identified at postmortem examination. This accounted for chronic renal failure.

CASE 20

Signalment: 6-year-old MC feline DSH

History: Approximately 1 month's duration of intermittent weakness, exercise intolerance, poor hair coat.

Physical Examination: Cat is near collapse and approximately 10% dehydrated. There is definite cervical ventroflexion.

Hematology		Reference Range
PCV (%)	41.0	24–45
NCC (×10³/μl)		
Segs (×10³/μl)	**18.0**	2.5–12.5
Monos (×10³/μl	0.7	0–0.8
Lymphs (×10³/μl)	**0.5**	1.5–7.0
Platelets (×10³/μl)	Adequate	150–700

Biochemical Profile		Reference Range
Gluc (mg/dl)	98	67–124
BUN (mg/dl)	**68 (24.3)**	17–32 (6.1–11.4 mmol/L)
Creat (mg/dl)	**2.8 (247)**	0.9–2.1 (80–186 μmol/L)
Ca (mg/dl)	10.9	8.5–11
Phos (mg/dl)	6.8	3.3–7.8
TP (g/dl)	**9.3**	5.9–8.1
Alb (g/dl)	**5.3**	2.3–3.9
Glob (g/dl)	4.0	2.9–4.4
T. Bili (mg/dl)	0.3	0–0.3
Chol (mg/dl)	180	60–220
ALT (IU/L)	52	30–100
ALP (IU/L)	48	6–106
CK (IU/L)	**2419**	60–300
Na (mEq/L)	157	146–160
K (mEq/L)	**2.0**	3.7–5.4
CL (mEq/L)	114	112–129
T CO₂ (mEq/L)	15	14–23
An. gap (mEq/L)	**30**	10–27

Blood Gas Data (arterial)		Reference Range
pH	**7.130**	7.33–7.44
PCO₂ (mmHg)	**44.0**	35–42
HCO₃ (mEq/L)	**14.0**	16–22

Urinalysis			
Color	Yellow	**Urine Sediment**	
Transparency	Cloudy	WBCs/hpf	0–2
Sp. Gr.	**1.014**	RBCs/hpf	0–2
Protein	Trace	Epith cells/hpf	0–2
Gluc	Negative	Casts/lpf	Negative
Bilirubin	Negative	Crystals	Negative
Blood	Negative	Bacteria	Negative
pH	5.5	Other	

Fractional excretion		Reference Range
Na (%)	0.55	<1.0
K (%)	**37.7**	<20.0

Interpretive Discussion

Hematology

There is a mature neutrophilia and lymphopenia, indicating a stress leukogram. Other components of the hemogram are normal.

Biochemical Profile

The BUN and serum creatinine concentrations are mildly increased. These findings are consistent with decreased glomerular filtration rate. However, one cannot differentiate the nature of the azotemia (prerenal, renal, or postrenal) based on these findings alone. Refer to the discussion of urinalysis results for further interpretation. The normal serum phosphorus and total calcium concentrations do not contribute to the characterization of renal disease.

Serum total protein and albumin concentrations are increased; this documents marked dehydration or hemoconcentration.

Serum CK activity is increased significantly and is indicative of muscle damage.

Serum Na and Cl concentrations are normal, but serum K concentration is markedly decreased. This is especially significant in light of the acidosis, which results in a shift of potassium from within cells to extracellular fluid and suggests a marked potassium deficit.

Blood Gas Data

There is prominent acidosis. This is due to a combined metabolic (decreased HCO_3) and respiratory (increased pCO_2) acidosis, with an increased anion gap. It would not be unusual for this degree of dehydration to lead to hypovolemia-induced lactic acidosis. It is also possible that this degree of hypokalemia may have caused sufficient respiratory muscle dysfunction to impair normal ventilation.

Urinalysis

The urinary specific gravity is in the isosthenuric range. Given the azotemia and normal serum Na and Cl concentrations, this indicates probable renal disease. However, hypokalemia can also impair ADH responsiveness by the kidneys, so that urine concentration should be evaluated following rehydration and K repletion.

The urinary FE_{Na} is 0.55%, which speaks against a generalized renal tubular disease. However, the FE_K is 37.7%, which is markedly increased, especially for a cat with this degree of hypokalemia.

Summary

The combined observations of azotemia, hypokalemia, acidosis, and hyperkaluria in a cat with cervical ventroflexion and evidence of widespread muscle damage support a diagnosis of feline kaliopenic polymyopathy/ nephropathy syndrome. In this case, it was completely corrected by dietary change (non-acidifying, higher K diet). This syndrome is no longer seen, as dietary imbalances in commercial cat food were corrected.

CASE 21

Signalment: 2-year-old male canine, West Highland white terrier
History: Polyuria, polydipsia

Hematology		Reference Range
PCV (%)	**33.0**	37–55
Hgb (g/dl)	**11.3**	12–18
RBC (×10⁶/µl)	**4.45**	5.5–8.5
MCV (fl)	**74.0**	60–72
MCHC (g/dl)	35.0	34–38
NCC (×10³/µl)	5.9	6–17
Segs (×10³/µl)	3.9	3–11.5
Monos (×10³/µl)	0.4	0.1–1.3
Lymphs (×10³/µl)	1.2	1–4.8
NRBC (×10³/µl)	**0.4**	0
Platelets (×10³/µl)	425	200–500
TP (P) (g/dl)	6.7	6–8

Hemopathology: Few acanthocytes and schistocytes

Biochemical Profile		Reference Range
Gluc (mg/dl)	108	65–122
BUN (mg/dl)	**65 (23.2)**	7–28 (2.5–10.0 mmol/L)
Creat (mg/dl)	**2.0 (176.8)**	0.9–1.7 (79–150 µmol/L)
Ca (mg/dl)	**7.2 (1.8)**	9.0–11.2 (2.25–2.8 mmol/L)
Phos (mg/dl)	6.1	2.8–6.1
TP (g/dl)	5.8	5.4–7.4
Alb (g/dl)	3.7	2.7–4.5
Glob (g/dl)	2.1	1.9–3.4
T. Bili (mg/dl)	0.3	0–0.4
Chol (mg/dl)	**382 (9.9)**	130–370 (3.4–9.6 mmol/L)
ALT (IU/L)	56	10–120
ALP (IU/L)	137	35–280
Na (mEq/L)	147	145–158
K (mEq/L)	**3.0**	4.1–5.5
CL (mEq/L)	115	106–127
TCO₂ (mEq/L)	22.3	14–27
An. gap (mEq/L)	12.7	8–25
Calc. Osmolality (mOsm/kg)	**317**	290–310

Blood Gas Data (arterial)		Reference Range
pH	7.349	7.33–7.45
PO₂ (mmHg)	80.1	67–92
PCO₂ (mmHg)	39.1	24–39
HCO₃ (mEq/L)	21.0	14–24
ionized Ca++ (mEq/L)	**3.44**	4.5–5.6

Urinalysis			
Color	Yellow	**Urine Sediment**	
Transparency	Clear	WBCs/hpf	3–6
Sp. Gr.	1.028	RBCs/hpf	3–6
Protein	**2+**	Epith cells/hpf	0–2
Gluc	**3+**	Casts/lpf	**Rare fine gran**
Bilirubin	1+	Crystals	Negative
Blood	Negative	Bacteria	Negative
pH	5.0		
ketones	Trace		
osmolality	358 (mOsm/L)		
UPC	**1.75**		

Fractional excretion		Reference Range
Na (%)	**1.62**	<1.0
Ca (%)	**7.47**	<1.0

Interpretive Discussion

Hematology

The packed cell volume, erythrocyte count, and hemoglobin concentration are decreased, indicating an anemia. Observed red blood cell morphologic abnormalities include acanthocytes and schistocytes. These may be observed when there is erythrocytic membrane damage due to free radical or lipid metabolic abnormalities, or when there is microangiopathic pathology due to vascular disease or neoplasia. Although a reticulocyte count has not been provided, the increased erythrocyte MCV and nucleated erythrocytes are consistent with a regenerative response. There are no other hematologic abnormalities.

Biochemical Profile

Serum glucose concentration is normal, and its importance in the interpretation of the glucosuria is discussed below.

The BUN and serum creatinine concentrations are increased, while the serum phosphorus value is at the upper limit of the reference range. These findings are consistent with decreased glomerular filtration rate. However, one cannot differentiate the nature of the azotemia (prerenal, renal, or postrenal) based on these findings alone. Refer to the discussion of urinalysis results for further interpretation.

The serum total calcium concentration is decreased. This does not correct to a normal value when adjusted for the serum albumin or total protein values. The ionized calcium concentration reported with the blood gas panel is likewise less than normal, indicating a true hypocalcemia.

Serum total protein, albumin, and globulin concentrations are within the reference range. This observation suggests that there is not hemoconcentration due to dehydration, although a concurrent protein-losing disorder might exist. Thus, the azotemia noted above is less likely due to dehydration, and more likely renal in origin.

Serum cholesterol is increased, whereas other indices of hepatic function are normal. There are no other indicators of a primary metabolic disease like diabetes mellitus, but it is possible, nevertheless, that this dog has hypothyroidism or hyperadrenocorticism.

The serum sodium and chloride concentrations are normal, yet there is hypokalemia. Possible causes in this case might include hyperadrenocorticism, chronic renal disease, or urinary potassium wasting associated with diuresis. Calculated serum osmolality is mildly increased due to the azotemia.

Blood Gas Data

Indices of acid-base metabolism (pH, pCO_2, HCO_3, and anion gap) are normal.

Urinalysis

Although the urinary specific gravity indicates concentrating ability, one might expect this to be greater if the azotemia were pre-renal in origin. It is also possible for the specific gravity to be increased by the presence of solutes which do not contribute to renal concentration capacity (glucose, protein, amino acids). Concomitant determination of urinary osmolality (358 mOsm/L) indicates that the urine is not being concentrated relative to the calculated osmolality of the serum. Inability to concentrate the urine may be due to central diabetes insipidus (a defect in hypothalamic/pituitary antidiuretic hormone release), or nephrogenic diabetes insipidus (ADH is released, but the kidney is unable to respond). The latter may be caused by anatomic pathology or functional impairment of renal tubular actions necessary to maintain a medullary concentration gradient and water reabsorption. This finding may indicate that the observed azotemia is renal in origin.

The presence of proteinuria on the dipstick was followed by a chemical determination of urinary protein concentration. When indexed to the urinary creatinine value, the urinary protein:creatinine ratio is 1.75. While this value is probably abnormal, it is not sufficiently high to indicate glomerular protein loss. Values in the range of 1.0 to 2.0 have been associated epidemiologically with tubular or inflammatory causes of proteinuria. The absence of significant numbers of leukocytes suggests there is no inflammatory disease. The presence of fine granular casts is indicative of renal tubular damage, and may explain the proteinuria.

Glucosuria concomitant to euglycemia may be explained by three mechanisms. (1) There is a Fanconi's-type syndrome wherein tubular malfunction leads to loss of glucose, protein, and other solutes which would otherwise be reabsorbed from the glomerular filtrate. This is supported by the findings of modest proteinuria and increased urinary fractional excretion of electrolytes. Fanconi's syndromes may be inherited (as reported in Basenjis and Whippets) or acquired (as reported following exposure to nephrotoxicants, including aminoglycoside antibiotics and heavy metals). (2) There was an earlier episode of hyperglycemia which exceeded the renal threshold for glucose reabsorption, during which time the urine analyzed was produced. Depending on the rate of urine formation, a single void may represent blood chemistry-related changes for many hours prior to specimen collection. (3) A laboratory error was made in the determination of either the serum glucose (improper preservation of the blood sample or analytical error) or the urinary glucose (cross-contamination of dipstick reaction squares by excess urine or operator error in interpreting the color change).

The FE_{Na} is 1.62%. This may be indicative of renal tubular disease or dysfunction due to mineralocorticoid deficiency or transport malfunction. The FE_{Ca} is 7.47%. This is particularly inappropriate given the hypocalcemia, and may well be the cause of calcium loss from the body. This may be indicative of renal tubular disease or dysfunction due to parathyroid hormone deficiency or transport malfunction. Increased urinary excretion of both of these electrolytes may be observed in renal failure (consider the azotemia and impaired urinary concentrating ability) or in Fanconi's syndrome, wherein proximal renal tubule reabsorptive function is impaired (consider the euglycemic glucosuria).

Summary

This is a case of congenital Fanconi's syndrome which did not resolve following supportive treatment for renal failure. Other tests one should perform include those that evaluate the parathyroid gland.

CASE 22

Signalment: 8-year-old male canine
History: Polydipsia
Physical Examination: Slightly dehydrated

Hematology		Reference Range
PCV (%)	38.0	37–55
Hgb (g/dl)	12.0	12–18
RBC (×10⁶/µl)	5.51	5.5–8.5
MCV (fl)	69.0	60–72
NCC (×10³/µl)	18.2	6–17
Segs (×10³/µl)	2.0	3–11.5
Monos (×10³/µl)	0.6	0.1–1.3
Lymphs (×10³/µl)	13.8	1–4.8
Platelets (×10³/µl)	298	200–500
TP (P) (g/dl)	8.8	6–8

Hemopathology: clumped platelets

Biochemical Profile		Reference Range
Gluc (mg/dl)	91	65–122
BUN (mg/dl)	33 (11.8)	7–28 (2.5–10.0 mmol/L)
Creat (mg/dl)	2.9 (256)	0.9–1.7 (80–150 µmol/L)
Ca (mg/dl)	15.4 (3.85)	9.0–11.2 (2.25–2.80 mmol/L)
Phos (mg/dl)	7.1 (2.3)	2.8–6.1 (0.9–2.0 mmol/L)
TP (g/dl)	7.9	5.4–7.4
Alb (g/dl)	4.0	2.7–4.5
Glob (g/dl)	3.9	1.9–3.4
T. Bili (mg/dl)	1.0 (17)	0–0.4 (0–6.8 µmol/L)
Chol (mg/dl)	291	130–370
ALT (IU/L)	152	10–120
AST (IU/L)	64	16–40
ALP (IU/L)	361	35–280
GGT (IU/L)	14	0–6
Na (mEq/L)	154	145–158
K (mEq/L)	5.8	4.1–5.5
CL (mEq/L)	109	106–127
TCO₂ (mEq/L)	12.1	14–27
An. gap (mEq/L)	38.7	8–25

Urinalysis			
Color	Straw	**Urine Sediment**	
Transparency	Clear	WBCs/hpf	2–3
Sp. Gr.	1.011	RBCs/hpf	1–2
Protein	2+	Epith cells/hpf	Negative
Gluc	Negative	Casts/lpf	Negative
Bilirubin	2+	Crystals	Negative
Blood	Negative	Bacteria	Negative
pH	6.5		
UPC	2.6		

Fractional excretion		Reference Range
Na (%)	1.73	<1.0
Ca (%)	3.37	<1.0

Interpretive Discussion

Hematology

The nucleated cell count is mildly increased, but there is a neutropenia and marked lymphocytosis. Other hematologic parameters, including cell morphology, are normal. However, the concurrent observation of marked lymphocytosis and neutropenia should alert one to the possibility of lymphocytic leukemia or lymphoma with bone marrow involvement or ehrlichiosis. The concurrent observation of marked lymphocytosis and hypercalcemia should likewise lead to consideration of lymphoma and humoral hypercalcemia of malignancy.

Biochemical Profile

The serum glucose concentration is normal.

The BUN, creatinine, and phosphorus concentrations are mildly increased. These findings are consistent with decreased glomerular filtration rate. However, one cannot differentiate the nature of the azotemia (pre-renal, renal, or post-renal) based on these findings alone. Refer to the discussion of urinalysis results for further interpretation.

The serum total calcium concentration is markedly increased. Common causes include hypercalcemia of malignancy.

The serum total protein and globulin concentrations are slightly increased. Increased globulin concentration may occur in dogs with lymphoproliferative disorders.

Serum cholesterol is normal in concentration. The total bilirubin concentration is increased, as are the serum ALP and GGT activities. These findings are evidence of cholestasis. There are mild increases in the serum activities of ALT and AST, so there may be some hepatocellular damage as well.

The increase in serum potassium is probably due to redistribution of intracellular potassium to extracellular potassium secondary to acidosis. The serum total CO_2 concentration is mildly decreased, indicating a metabolic acidosis. A complete blood gas panel is required to completely evaluate acid-base status.

Urinalysis

The urine specific gravity is in the isosthenuric range. The dog does not appear to be dehydrated, and it is possible for a normal dog to produce urine with a specific gravity in this range. However, the concurrent observation of azotemia is indicative of renal dysfunction, and the concurrent observation of hypercalcemia may represent calcium antagonism of antidiuretic hormone (ADH) activity. There is significant proteinuria of 2+ on the dipstick, and a UPC of 2.6. In the absence of significant sediment changes, this is indicative of renal protein loss, probably glomerular in origin. The FE_{Na} is 1.73%, indicating tubular dysfunction. Thus, the combination of azotemia, isosthenuria, proteinuria, and natriuria all support a diagnosis of renal disease.

Summary

This is a case of lymphoma with hypercalcemia of malignancy and hypercalcemic nephropathy.

CASE 23

Signalment: 9-year-old female dog
History: Polydipsia, polyuria
Physical Examination: Mass in pelvic inlet

Biochemical Profile		Reference Range
Gluc (mg/dl)	106	65–122
BUN (mg/dl)	8	7–28
Creat (mg/dl)	1.4	0.9–1.7
TP (g/dl)	**7.7**	5.4–7.4
Alb (g/dl)	**5.2**	2.7–4.5
Ca (mg/dl)	**16.4 (4.5)**	9.0–11.2 (2.25–2.80 mmol/L)
Phos (mg/dl)	3.5	2.8–6.1
T. Bili (mg/dl)	0.2	0–0.4
ALT (IU)	43	10–120
ALP (IU)	**428**	35–280
Na (mEq/L)	155	145–158
K (mEq/L)	3.9	4.1–5.5
CL (mEq/L)	119	106–127
TCO$_2$ (mEq/L)	21.6	14–27

Urinalysis	
Urine specific gravity	**1.014**

Interpretive Discussion

Biochemical Profile

There is marked hypercalcemia and this magnitude of increase is suggestive of hypercalcemia of malignancy or primary hyperparathyroidism. Hypercalcemia of this magnitude would be expected to result in renal injury leading to azotemia and loss of concentrating ability. The concentration ability may be impaired, because the urine specific gravity is nearly isosthenuric. This interpretation is supported by the observation of polyuria; however, hypercalcemia may interfere with activity.

A moderate increase in alkaline phosphatase activity ADH indicates cholestasis or previous treatment with corticosteroids. The normal serum bilirubin suggests cholestosis is not present. An alternate explanation for the increased alkaline phosphatase might be increased bone turnovers secondary to increased serum concentration of PTH or PTHrp.

Summary

The mass in the pelvis was aspirated, and appeared neuroendocrine, rather than lymphoid. At surgery, the mass was removed and confirmed by histopathology to be a perirectal apocrine gland adenocarcinoma. Following surgery, the calcium normalized, but some time later metastasis to the lungs resulted in return of hypercalcemia. In contrast to the previous case, the hypercalcemia has not yet resulted in sufficient renal injury to cause azotemia.

CASE 24

Signalment: 6-month-old DSH female cat
History: Vomiting, weakness, acute onset
Physical Examination: Tachypnea for 24 hours, weakness

Hematology		Reference Range
PCV (%)	40	24–45
WBC (×10³/µl)	**21.0**	5500–19500
Segs (×10³/µl)	**20.2**	2500–12500
Bands (×10³/µl)	0	0–300
Lymphs (×10³/µl)	**0.2**	1500–7000
Monos (×10³/µl)	0.6	0–850

Biochemical Profile		Reference Range
Gluc (mg/dl)	**150 (8.2)**	67–124 (3.7–6.8 mmol/L)
BUN (mg/dl)	**45 (16.1)**	17–32 (6.1–11.4 mmol/L)
Creat (mg/dl)	**2.2 (194)**	0.9–2.1 (80–186 µmol/L)
Ca (mg/dl)	**18 (4.5)**	8.5–11 (2.12–2.75 mmol/L)
Phos (mg/dl)	**9.5 (3.1)**	3.3–7.8 (1.1–2.5 mmol/L)
TP (g/dl)	8.0	5.9–8.1
Alb (g/dl)	**4.2**	2.3–3.9
Glob (g/dl)	3.8	2.9–4.4
T. Bili (mg/dl)	0.2	0–0.3
Chol (mg/dl)	120	60–270
ALT (IU)	100	30–100
ALP (IU)	25	11–210
Na (mEq/L)	159	146–160
K (mEq/L)	**6.4**	3.7–5.4
CL (mEq/L)	112	112–129
TCO₂ (mEq/L)	16.8	14–24
An. gap (mEq/L)	37	10–27

Blood Gas Data (arterial)		Reference Range
pH	**6.926**	7.33–7.44
PCO₂ (mmHg)	**72.1**	35–42
PO₂ (mmHg)	**65**	80–95
HCO₃ (mEq/L)	**14.9**	16–22

Urinalysis	
Sp. Gr.	1.020
Gran casts/hpf	2

Interpretive Discussion

Hematology

There is a stress leukogram indicated by mature neutrophilia and lymphopenia.

Biochemical Profile

Increased glucose is compatible with stress identified in the leukogram. The BUN and creatinine are mildly increased, indicating azotemia. The urine specific gravity is less than what one would expect in a cat with prerenal azotemia, therefore renal azotemia should be considered. With a calcium of 18 mg/dl, renal dysfunction is likely occurring due to soft tissue mineralization. The total protein and albumin are increased, particularly for a young cat, indicating dehydration.

The calcium is markedly increased. Primary causes of this degree of hypercalcemia are hypercalcemia of malignancy, primary hyperparathyroidism, and hypervitaminosis D. Vitamin D toxicosis should be very high on the differential list, due to the age of the cat and the acute onset. Because of acidosis, ionized calcium is likely very high. Phosphorus is mildly increased. This could be in part due to the young age of the cat or may be due to decreased GFR. It is also seen with hypervitaminosis D. The CaxP product is markedly increased at 171, which will result in calcification of renal tubules, lungs and other soft tissues.

Potassium is increased. This may be due to acidosis and an associated shift of K out of cells or the animal may be becoming oliguric. The total CO_2 is borderline low, indicating a component of metabolic acidosis. Increased anion gap indicates increase in unmeasured anions. Possible unmeasured anions are lactic acid or uremic acids. Increased phosphates are also adding to the anion gap.

Blood Gas Data

The pH is extremely decreased indicating severe acidosis. The pCO_2 is the major abnormality in the balance between bicarbonate and CO_2. Therefore, respiratory acidosis is the major component of the acidosis. The bicarbonate is also decreased indicating a component of metabolic acidosis is superimposed. Hypoxemia is also present. The combined hypoxemia and retention of CO_2 indicate a severe ventilation abnormality, probably due to calcification of lungs. The metabolic acidosis is probably a result of renal failure.

Summary

The cat was diagnosed with renal disease with severe acidemia, both metabolic and respiratory. The respiratory component may be due to calcification of lungs. Cholecalciferol toxicosis was diagnosed, as the cat had an opportunity to ingest a rodenticide containing cholecalciferol.

CASE 25

Signalment: 3-year-old male cat
History: Acute lethargy, vomiting, and anorexia
Physical Examination: Obese, almost comatose

Hematology		Reference Range
PCV (%)	50	24–45
NCC (×10³/µl)	25.0	5.5–19.5
Segs (×10³/µl)	23.0	2.5–12.5
Monos (×10³/µl)	1.7	0–0.88
Lymphs (×10³/µl)	0.3	1.5–7.0
Platelets (×10³/µl)	Adequate	150–700

Biochemical Profile		Reference Range
Gluc (mg/dl)	285	67–124
BUN (mg/dl)	110	17–32
Creat (mg/dl)	7.5	0.9–2.1
Ca (mg/dl)	6.5	8.5–11
Phos (mg/dl)	14	3.3–7.8
TP (g/dl)	9.0	5.9–8.1
Alb (g/dl)	4.9	2.3–3.9
Glob (g/dl)	4.1	2.9–4.4
T. Bili (mg/dl)	0.3	0–0.3
ALT (IU)	35	30–100
ALP (IU)	45	11–210
Na (mEq/L)	165	146–160
K (mEq/L)	6.8	3.7–5.4
CL (mEq/L)	107	112–129
TCO₂ (mEq/L)	10	14–23
An. gap (mEq/L)	55	10–27
Calc. Osmolality (mOsm/kg)	394	290–310
Meas. Osmolality (mOsm/kg)	440	290–310
Osmolal Gap (mOsm/kg)	46	>10

Urinalysis (cystocentesis)			
Color	Yellow	**Urine Sediment**	
Transparency	Cloudy	WBCs/hpf	2–3
Sp. Gr.	1.016	RBCs/hpf	2–3
Protein	1+	Epith cells/hpf	1–3 transitional
Gluc	1+	Casts/lpf	0
Bilirubin	Negative	Crystals	**Calcium oxalate (monohydrate)**
Blood	1+	Bacteria	0
pH	5.0		

Interpretive Discussion

Hematology

PCV is slightly increased. This is likely due to dehydration, considering that the albumin is also increased. The mature neutrophilia and lymphopenia are suggestive of a stress or corticosteroid leukogram.

Biochemical Profile

The serum glucose concentration is increased. Differentials should include stress or corticosteroids, excitement and diabetes mellitus. Excitement is less likely than the others, since the cat does not have an excitement leukogram. (See summary for further discussion of hyperglycemia.)

The BUN and creatinine are increased, and considering that the cat is not concentrating its urine, this is most likely a renal azotemia. Since the cat is dehydrated, a prerenal component to the azotemia may be present as well. Because the cat is not anemic, is obese, and the history is acute, this is most likely acute renal failure. Phosphorus is increased due to decreased glomerular filtration rate.

The serum calcium is decreased. Considering that the cat likely has acute renal failure, the most likely cause of the hypocalcemia is formation of calcium oxalate crystals associated with ethylene glycol toxicosis. Oxalate is one of the metabolites of ethylene glycol and combines with calcium to form calcium oxalate crystals.

The serum total protein and concentration is increased due to dehydration, since hyperalbuminemia is present.

The sodium is increased, likely due to dehydration. Hyperkalemia suggests oliguria or anuria and is also partially due to intracellular to extracellular redistribution secondary to acidosis. Serum total CO_2 is decreased, suggesting metabolic acidosis. The metabolites of ethylene glycol are acids, and cause metabolic acidosis.

The increased anion gap indicates increased concentrations of anions other than those used in the formula to calculate the anion gap (chloride and HCO_3^-). In this case, uremic acid, phosphate, albumin, and most importantly, metabolites of ethylene glycol are probably contributing to the anion gap. Chloride and HCO_3^- (TCO_2) is a result of accumulation of these other anions (high anion gap metabolic acidosis).

The calculated osmolality is increased, since the substances that are included in the formula to calculate osmolality are increased (glucose, urea, sodium, potassium). However, the actual plasma osmolality is much higher than the calculated osmolality, since a substance is present in the blood that is not used in the formula to calculate osmolality. The most common cause of an increased osmole gap is the presence of ethylene glycol, which contributes to plasma osmolality due to its low molecular weight.

Urinalysis

The urine specific gravity of 1.016 in an azotemic dehydrated cat indicates that the cat is not capable of concentrating urine, and that renal dysfunction is present. The presence of calcium oxalate crystals in a cat with acute renal failure is very suggestive of ethylene glycol toxicosis. The renal threshold for glucose has been exceeded, resulting in glucosuria. The 1+ proteinurea is probably significant in light of the low urine specific gravity and probably resulted from tubular damage.

Summary

The cat died, and necropsy revealed renal tubular necrosis and the presence of calcium oxalate crystals in the tubules due to ethylene glycol toxicosis. The cat had access to antifreeze shortly before it became ill. Approximately 50% of dogs and cats with ethylene glycol induced renal failure have hyperglycemia, probably due to a combination of stress and the formation of aldehyde, a metabolite of ethylene glycol that interferes with glucose metabolism. While diabetes mellitus could cause hyperglycemia and metabolic acidosis, the presence of acute renal failure and calcium oxalate crystalluria should be very suggestive of ethylene glycol toxicosis.

CASE 26

Signalment: 3-month-old Saint Bernard
History: Stumbling for 4 hours
Physical Examination: Cannot stand, in a stupor
Hematology: No abnormalities.

Biochemical Profile		Reference Range
Gluc (mg/dl)	**129**	65–122
BUN (mg/dl)	20	7–28
Creat (mg/dl)	1.6	0.9–1.7
Ca (mg/dl)	11.2	9.0–11.2
Ionized calcium (mg/dl)	5.6	4.5–5.6
Phos (mg/dl)	**10.2**	2.8–6.1
TP (g/dl)	5.8	5.4–7.4
Alb (g/dl)	2.9	2.7–4.5
Glob (g/dl)	2.4	1.9–3.4
T. Bili (mg/dl)	0.2	0–0.4
Chol (mg/dl)	220	130–370
ALT (IU/L)	60	10–120
AST (IU/L)	30	16–40
ALP (IU/L)	**300**	35–280
GGT (IU/L)	2	0–6
Na (mEq/L)	148	145–158
K (mEq/L)	5.2	4.1–5.5
CL (mEq/L)	105	106–127
HCO$_3$ (mEq/L)	15.1	14–27
An. gap (mEq/L)	**33**	8–25
Meas. Osmolality (mOsm/kg)	**442**	290–310
Calc. Osmolality (mOsm/kg)	**330**	290–310
Osmole gap (mOsm/kg)	**112**	0–10
Serum ethylene glycol concentration (mg/dl)	**>250**	0

Blood Gas Data (arterial)		Reference Range
Blood pH	7.305	7.24–7.50
HCO$_3$ (mEq/L)	**13.7**	15–24
PCO$_2$ (mm/Hg)	29	26–39

Urinalysis	
Urine specific gravity	**1.012**
Urine pH	5

Interpretive Discussion

Biochemical Profile

The serum glucose concentration is slightly increased. This may be due to stress, although the leukogram is nor-mal. Aldehydes, a metabolite of ethylene glycol, are re-ported to interfere with glucose metabolism.

The BUN and creatinine are normal in this dog that has a high serum ethylene glycol concentration. In dogs, azotemia begins between 24 and 36 hours following in-gestion. The history suggests that this dog ingested anti-freeze approximately 5 hours prior to the time of these laboratory data.

Phosphorus is markedly increased. Hyperphospha-temia may be due to the young age of the dog, but is somewhat high for this. In this case the serum phospho-rus increase was likely due to phosphate rust inhibitors present in most commercial antifreeze.

Serum alkaline phosphatase activity is mildly increased, likely due to the bone isoenzyme that is increased in grow-ing dogs.

The anion gap is increased, likely due to either phos-phates or metabolites of ethylene glycol, which are an-ions. The calculated osmolality is slightly increased. However, the actual plasma osmolality is much higher than the calculated osmolality, resulting in a large os-mole gap, since a substance is present in the blood that is not used in the formula to calculate osmolality. The most common cause of an increased osmole gap is the presence of ethylene glycol, which contributes to plasma osmolal-ity due to its low molecular weight. This was confirmed by measuring serum ethylene glycol concentration.

Blood Gas Data

The HCO$_3$ is decreased, indicating metabolic acidosis. Metabolites of ethylene glycol are acids. The blood gases were determined about one hour following the biochem-ical profile, which probably accounts for the discrepancy between the HCO$_3$ determined on the biochemical panel, and that from the blood gas machine.

Urinalysis

The urine specific gravity of 1.012 in this patient is likely due to ethylene glycol causing osmotic diuresis. It is also possible that concentrating ability has been im-paired, but the animal is not yet azotemic.

Summary

The dog was treated with fomepizole, an alcohol dehy-drogenase inhibitor, approximately 7 to 8 hours following antifreeze ingestion, and did not become azotemic. In con-trast to the previous case, the biochemical profile is often not diagnostic in acute ethylene glycol poisoning, and other tests, such as serum ethylene glycol concentration or mea-sured osmolality must be used to confirm the diagnosis. The acute onset of stumbling and stupor triggered suspi-cion of ethylene glycol toxicosis.

CASE 27

Signalment: 6-day-old female Holstein
History: Scours
Physical Examination: Severe dehydration

Hematology		Reference Range
PCV (%)	**58.0**	24–46
Hgb (g/dl)	**19.0**	8–15
RBC (×10⁶/μl)	**17.1**	5.0–10.0
MCV (fl)	**34.0**	37–53
MCHC (g/dl)	33.0	34–38
NCC (×10³/μl)	5.0	4.0–12.0
Segs (×10³/μl)	3.2	0.6–4.0
Monos (×10³/μl)	**1.7**	0–0.8
Lymphs (×10³/μl)	**0.1**	2.5–7.5
Platelets (×10³/μl)	288	200–800
Fibrinogen (mg/dl)	600	200–600
TP (P) (g/dl)	**10.9**	6–8

Hemopathology: many acanthocytes and keratocytes, RBC fragments, hypochromic RBCs.

Biochemical Profile		Reference Range
Gluc (mg/dl)	**31**	55–95
BUN (mg/dl)	**87**	7–20
Creat (mg/dl)	**4.6**	1.0–1.8
Ca (mg/dl)	**7.8**	8.2–9.9
Phos (mg/dl)	6.9	4.3–7.0
TP (g/dl)	**10.3**	6.3–7.6
Alb (g/dl)	**5.3**	2.5–4.3
Glob (g/dl)	**5.0**	2.6–5.0
T. Bili (mg/dl)	**0.8**	0.1–0.4
CK (IU/L)	**352**	57–280
AST (IU/L)	**286**	40–130
GGT (IU/L)	14	10–26
SDH (IU/L)	17	8–23
Na (mEq/L)	**129**	136–147
K (mEq/L)	**6.7**	3.6–5.2
CL (mEq/L)	**91**	95–105
TCO₂ (mEq/L)	**17.0**	24–32
An. gap (mEq/L)	**27.7**	14–26

Blood Gas Data (venous)		Reference Range
pH	**7.140**	7.32–7.45
pCO₂ (mmHg)	**45.7**	34–44
HCO₃ (mEq/L)	**15.3**	23–31

Urinalysis				
Color	Yellow	**Urine Sediment**		
Transparency	Clear	WBCs/hpf	0–1	
Sp. Gr.	1.014	RBCs/hpf	0–1	
Protein	Negative	Epith cells/hpf	1–2	
Gluc	Negative	Casts/lpf	Negative	
Bilirubin	Negative	Crystals	Negative	
Blood	Negative	Bacteria	Negative	
pH	5.0			

Interpretive Discussion

Hematology

There is a monocytosis and a lymphopenia that represent the effects of stress. The plasma protein concentration is increased, most probably due to dehydration. Erythrocyte indices reflect hemoconcentration as well, as evidenced by the increased RBC count, hemoglobin concentration, and PCV. The MCV and MCHC are decreased, which may be due to an underlying iron-deficiency anemia of the newborn, which is obscured by hemoconcentration. The presence of several erythrocyte morphologic abnormalities supports this possibility. Iron deficiency is frequently associated not only with a microcytic anemia, but also with oxidative damage to the erythrocytes, resulting in membrane abnormalities and fragmentation changes.

Biochemical Profile

There is a profound hypoglycemia, which in a neonatal calf with diarrhea is most probably related to decreased food intake, as well as the possibility of sepsis. Sepsis is unlikely, considering the normal neutrophil concentration.

The BUN and serum creatinine concentrations are increased, but the origin of this azotemia cannot be discerned from this data alone. Refer to the discussion or the urinalysis below.

Serum calcum is mildly decreased, possibly due to decreased milk intake. The serum total protein and albumin concentrations are increased, further reflecting hemoconcentration due to dehydration. The serum CK and AST activities are modestly increased, which may be related to muscle damage subsequent to prolonged recumbency or hypoperfusion. The total bilirubin is increased. Together with the increased AST activity, this may indicate hepatocellular damage. Alternatively, there may be cholestasis due to dehydration or prehepatic icterus due to increased destruction of oxidatively-damaged iron-deficient erythrocytes.

The serum sodium and chloride concentrations are decreased, reflecting decreased intake and/or increased loss from the body. *E. coli*-associated diarrhea in neonatal calves commonly results from increased sodium chloride loss induced by the enterotoxin that promotes active secretion into the gut lumen. Increased water loss follows this osmotic gradient. Bicarbonate is also lost in the feces, and hypovolemia may lead to tissue hypoperfusion, lactic acidosis, and decreased bicarbonate concentration as well. Fecal potassium loss is typically increased, but concomitant metabolic acidosis results in exchange of intracellular potassium for extracellular protons, and a redistributional hyperkalemia.

Blood Gas Data

There is a combined metabolic (decreased bicarbonate) and respiratory (increased pCO_2) acidosis. The metabolic acidosis results from bicarbonate loss in the diarrhea and from lactic acidosis due to tissue hypoperfusion. The increased anion gap reflects the accumulation of unmeasured anions such as lactate. The mild respiratory acidosis indicates pulmonary dysfunction. Early pneumonia or decreased pulmonary perfusion secondary to dehydration are possible explanations.

Urinalysis

The only significant abnormality is a urine specific gravity of 1.014. Six-day-old calves, unlike neonates of many other species, should have mature capacity to concentrate urine. Dehydration should stimulate antidiuretic hormone release from the hypothalamus, and increased water reclamation by the renal tubules. However, electrolyte loss in this type of hypotonic dehydration often leads to medullary solute depletion and a loss of the renal concentration gradient. Another alternative is that there is renal disease, due to renal hypoperfusion, sepsis, etc., resulting in both azotemia and loss of concentrating ability.

Summary

Secretory diarrhea and hypotonic dehydration in a neonatal calf.

CASE 28

Signalment: 9-month-old bull
History: Anorexia, depression
Physical Examination: Enlarged abdomen

Hematology		Reference Range
PCV (%)	19	24–46
MCV (fl)	31	37–53
NCC (×10³/µl)	18.0	4.0–12.0
Segs (×10³/µl)	10.5	0.6–4.0
Bands (×10³/µl)	2.5	0–0.1
Monos (×10³/µl)	1.0	0–0.8
Lymphs (×10³/µl)	3.5	2.5–7.5
Eos (×10³/µl)	0.5	0–2.4
Platelets (×10³/µl)	Adequate	200–800
Fibrinogen (mg/dl)	1000	200–600

Hemopathology: Numerous schistocytes, keratocytes

Biochemical Profile		Reference Range
Gluc (mg/dl)	618	55–95
BUN (mg/dl)	90	7–20
Creat (mg/dl)	6.1	1.0–1.8
Ca (mg/dl)	7.8	8.2–9.9
Phos (mg/dl)	14.1	4.3–7.0
TP (g/dl)	10.1	6.3–7.6
Alb (g/dl)	4.5	2.5–4.3
Glob (g/dl)	5.6	2.6–5.0
T. Bili (mg/dl)	0.8	0.1–0.4
CK (IU/L)	1100	57–280
AST (IU/L)	350	40–130
Na (mEq/L)	130	136–147
K (mEq/L)	3.1	3.6–5.2
CL (mEq/L)	47	95–105
TCO₂ (mEq/L)	50	24–32

Blood Gas Data (Venous)		Reference Range
HCO₃ (mEq/L)	49.3	23–31
pH	7.412	7.32–7.45
pCO₂ (mmHg)	80	34–44

Interpretive Discussion

Hematology

PCV is decreased, indicating anemia.

MCV is decreased, suggesting iron deficiency anemia secondary to chronic blood loss.

Neutrophilia, increased band neutrophils, and monocytosis are indicative of chronic inflammation.

Increased fibrinogen also suggests inflammation.

Keratocytes and schistocytes are commonly seen with iron deficiency anemia.

Biochemical Profile

Glucose is markedly increased, perhaps a sympatho-adrenal response that can be seen in severely ill cattle. Other possibilities include prior treatment with glucose-containing fluids, diabetes mellitus, or acute pancreatitis. Other lab data supports proximal duodenal obstruction, in which marked hyperglycemia is a consistent finding. This may be due to a combination of stress-induced hyperglycemia and poor peripheral perfusion, so that the glucose isn't used. Also low K may result in decreased cell uptake of glucose.

BUN, creatinine, and phosphorus are increased. Urine specific gravity would help determine if renal or pre-renal. Because of severe dehydration as indicated by increased albumin, at least a pre-renal component is likely. Phosphorus may also be increased due to high GI obstruction, which is likely the diagnosis.

Calcium slightly decreased. Phosphorus is excreted in the saliva of ruminants; with GI obstruction, elimination of phosphorus via the GI tract is decreased. Mild hypocalcemia has been reported with abomasal and forestomach disease.

Total protein and albumin are increased, indicating dehydration. Globulin is increased, which may be due to dehydration or antigenic stimulation.

Bilirubin is increased, which in this patient may be due to cholestasis or anorexia.

Serum creatine kinase activity is increased, probably indicative of myopathy. AST is mildly increased, either from myopathy or hepatocellular damage.

Marked hypochloremia is probably due to abomasal acid secretion into the lumen. Obstruction of abomasal out flow and distention exacerbates. Chloride is decreased more than would be expected with abomasal displacement or volvulus; this degree of hypochloremia is indicative of high GI obstruction. Potassium is likely decreased for the same reason.

Sodium is low and is perhaps being lost in urine. This may be due to hyperglycemia resulting in osmotic diuresis and thus increasing urinary losses of electrolytes.

Hyperosmolality may also be contributing to hyponatremia, as a result of cellular water moving into extracellular fluid compartment, diluting serum sodium (1.6 mEq/L decrease in Na for every 100 mg/dl increase in glucose)

Total CO_2 and HCO_3 are increased, indicating marked hypochloremic metabolic alkalosis. pH is in the high normal range as a result of compensatory respiratory acidosis (increased pCO_2). Remarkable hypochloremia and alkalosis indicated that there is obstruction of abomasal out flow, preventing re-exchange of chloride and bicarbonate.

Increased anion gap (36 mEq/L) also indicates increase in unmeasured anions. Most of the anions contributing to this are not truly "unmeasured," but are the increased phosphates and protein. Additionally, there may be increased lactate due to decreased tissue perfusion, or increased sulfates due to tissue breakdown.

Summary

This animal had a high GI obstruction (foreign body), thus explaining many of the abnormalities.

Azotemia was probably prerenal due to dehydration, although there are abnormalities in distal tubular transport which may be due to hypochloremia; osmotic diuresis may be also contributing to these abnormalities.

Inflammation is present, perhaps associated with the GI obstruction.

Iron deficiency anemia from chronic blood loss is present (perhaps abomasal ulcer, GI parasites).

Other tests that should be performed include urinalysis, especially specific gravity, and fecal occult blood.

CASE 29

Signalment: 9-day-old female Holstein
History: Several days duration of diarrhea, anorexia, extreme weakness
Physical Examination: Hypothermic, 12% dehydrated

Hematology		Reference Range
PCV (%)	51	24–46
NCC (×10³/µl)	19.7	4.0–12.0
Segs (×10³/µl)	11.4	0.6–4.0
Monos (×10³/µl)	2.0	0–0.8
Lymphs (×10³/µl)	6.3	2.5–7.5
Platelets (×10³/µl)	Adequate	200–800

Biochemical Profile		Reference Range
Gluc (mg/dl)	46	55–95
BUN (mg/dl)	63	7–20
Creat (mg/dl)	3.7	1.0–1.8
Ca (mg/dl)	5.9	8.2–9.9
Phos (mg/dl)	14.5	4.3–7.0
TP (g/dl)	3.0	6.3–7.6
Alb (g/dl)	1.9	2.5–4.3
Glob (g/dl)	1.1	2.6–5.0
T. Bili (mg/dl)	0.2	0.1–0.4
CK (IU/L)	7819	57–280
AST (IU/L)	177	40–130
GGT (IU/L)	28	10–26
Na (mEq/L)	158	136–147
K (mEq/L)	7.9	3.6–5.2
CL (mEq/L)	117	95–105
TCO₂ (mEq/L)	15	24–32
An. gap (mEq/L)	33.9	14–26

Blood Gas Data (Venous)		Reference Range
pH	7.140	7.32–7.45
pCO₂ (mmHg)	45.7	34–44
HCO₃ (mEq/L)	15.3	23–31

Interpretive Discussion

Hematology

There is a neutrophilia and monocytosis, indicating an inflammatory leukogram. The PCV is increased, reflecting hemoconcentration due to dehydration.

Biochemical Profile

There is a profound hypoglycemia, which in a neonatal calf with diarrhea is most probably related to decreased food intake, as well as the possibility of sepsis. Considering the increased neutrophil concentration, sepsis is unlikely.

The BUN and serum creatinine concentrations are increased, but the origin of this azotemia cannot be discerned without a urinalysis. However, given the other evidence of hemoconcentration, prerenal azotemia is the most likely cause. Although higher serum phosphorus concentrations are common in young animals, this degree of hyperphosphatemia is more likely related to decreased glomerular filtration rate. There is a marked hypocalcemia, but this may be due solely to the hypoalbuminemia; i.e., the ionized calcium concentration may be normal, but the protein-bound fraction is decreased.

There is marked hypoproteinemia, despite the severe degree of dehydration. This is due both to hypoalbuminemia and hypoglobulinemia. The former may be due to liver disease, inanition, or intestinal loss associated with the diarrhea. The latter is very likely due to lack of passive transfer, which would have subsequently predisposed this neonate to infections, resulting in diarrhea and sepsis.

The increased serum CK and AST activities may be due to muscle damage, to prolonged recumbency, or hypoperfusion. The very slight increase in GGT activity may be due to absorption of a small amount of colostrum, which is high in GGT activity in ruminants.

The increased serum sodium and chloride indicate that this calf is hypertonically dehydrated. One typically expects hypotonic dehydration to develop in a neonatal calf with scours, owing to electrolyte loss in the secretory diarrhea. Thus, it is more likely that this is not a secretory diarrhea, but rather another infectious cause of diarrhea, with or without septicemia. Water loss in excess of solute may be compounded by reduced water consumption, increased insensible losses due to fever, and/or exudation (along with albumin) across a damaged intestinal mucosa. Although there may have been significant potassium loss in the diarrhea, redistributional hyperkalemia is commonly observed in cases like this owing to exchange of intracellular potassium for extracellular protons (H^+) in response to the metabolic acidosis. The respiratory acidosis suggests inadequate pulmonary perfusion.

Blood Gas Data

There is a combined metabolic (decreased bicarbonate) and respiratory (increased pCO_2) acidosis. The metabolic acidosis results from bicarbonate loss in the diarrhea and from lactic acidosis due to tissue hypoperfusion. The increased anion gap reflects the accumulation of unmeasured anions like lactate.

Summary

Nonsecretory diarrhea and hypertonic dehydration in a neonatal calf following failure of passive transfer.

CASE 30

Signalment: 5-year-old spayed female Manx cat
History: Decreased appetite of approximately 2 weeks' duration. Fluid draining from a fistula over the terminal coccygeal vertebrae of 8 months' duration.
Physical Examination: Approximately 6% dehydrated. Coccygeal vertebrae were noted to terminate cranial to the anal sphincter. The fistula was noninflamed and draining a clear, colorless fluid.

Hematology		Reference Range
PCV (%)	**49**	24–45
NCC (×10³/µl)	11.6	5.5–19.5
Segs (×10³/µl)	9.6	2.5–12.5
Monos (×10³/µl)	0.6	0–0.8
Lymphs (×10³/µl)	**1.4**	1.5–7.0
Platelets (×10³/µl)	Adequate	150–700

Biochemical Profile		Reference Range
Gluc (mg/dl)	91	67–124
BUN (mg/dl)	**82**	17–32
Creat (mg/dl)	**2.2**	0.9–2.1
Ca (mg/dl)	**7.3**	8.5–11
Phos (mg/dl)	5.2	3.3–7.8
TP (g/dl)	**8.4**	5.9–8.1
Alb (g/dl)	**4.1**	2.3–3.9
Glob (g/dl)	4.3	2.9–4.4
T. Bili (mg/dl)	0.1	0–0.3
Chol (mg/dl)	153	60–220
ALT (IU/L)	40	30–100
Na (mEq/L)	**131**	146–160
K (mEq/L)	4.6	3.7–5.4
CL (mEq/L)	**101**	112–129
TCO₂ (mEq/L)	16	14–23
An. gap (mEq/L)	18.6	10–27

Urinalysis	
Color	Straw
Transparency	Clear
Sp. Gr.	**1.015**
Protein	Negative
Gluc	Negative
Bilirubin	Negative
Blood	Negative
pH	6.5

Fractional excretion		Reference Range
Na (%)	0.03	<1.0
CL (%)	0.08	<1.0

Interpretive Discussion

Hematology

The increased PCV is consistent with hemoconcentration due to dehydration. Other data are unremarkable.

Biochemical Profile

The azotemia (increased BUN and serum creatinine concentrations) may be prerenal and/or renal. Refer to the discussion of urinalysis below.

There is hypocalcemia, despite hyperproteinemia due to hemoconcentration, indicating that serum calcium concentration is truly decreased. This may have occurred secondary to chloride depletion and loss of the electrochemical gradient need to support calcium absorption from the glomerular filtrate in the Loop of Henle of the renal tubules.

Serum sodium and chloride are decreased in concentration. This usually reflects increased loss, compounded by reduced intake in sick, anorexic patients. In this case, there is physical evidence of cerebrospinal fluid loss from a draining meningomyelocele. Cerebrospinal fluid contains higher sodium and chloride concentrations than the blood, owing to the active chloride transport mechanism employed by the choroid plexus for secretion. Draining CSF from the body will create electrolyte depletion in excess of water, an otherwise classic scenario for hypotonic dehydration. Although this cat had been losing CSF for some time, the development of anorexia probably precipitated an imbalance between these pathologic losses and replacement of the electrolytes, resulting in the clinical presentation.

Urinalysis

The urinary fractional excretion values for sodium and chloride were well within the normal reference range, thereby ruling out renal loss as a cause for the electrolyte depletion. The only significant abnormality is a urine specific gravity of 1.015. Dehydration should stimulate antidiuretic hormone release form the hypothalamus, and increased water reclamation by the renal tubules. However, electrolyte loss in this type of hypotonic dehydration often leads to medullary solute depletion and a loss of the renal concentration gradient. Another alternative is that there is renal disease, due to renal hypoperfusion, sepsis, etc., resulting in both azotemia and loss of concentrating ability.

Summary

Sodium chloride depletion in a manx cat with a fistulated meningomyelocele (Hall JA, MJ Fettman, JT Ingram. Sodium chloride depletion in a cat with fistulated meningomyelocele. J Am Vet Med Assoc 1988;192: 1445–1448).

CASE 31

Signalment: 10-year-old female horse
History: Abdominal pain
Physical Examination: Tense abdomen, slight fever

Hematology		Reference Range
PCV (%)	52.0	32–52
Hgb (g/dl)	18.1	11–19
RBC (×10⁶/μl)	11.15	6.5–12.5
MCV (fl)	46.0	36–52
MCHC (g/dl)	34.0	34–39
NCC (×10³/μl)	14.2	5.5–12.5
Segs (×10³/μl)	11.8	2.7–6.7
Monos (×10³/μl)	0.3	0–0.8
Lymphs (×10³/μl)	2.1	1.5–5.5
Platelets (×10³/μl)	162	100–600
TP (P) (g/dl)	7.0	6–8

Biochemical Profile		Reference Range
Gluc (mg/dl)	166	70–110
BUN (mg/dl)	23	14–27
Creat (mg/dl)	4.2	1.1–2.0
Ca (mg/dl)	10.5	11.0–13.7
Phos (mg/dl)	4.5	1.9–4.1
TP (g/dl)	7.1	5.8–7.6
Alb (g/dl)	3.2	2.7–3.7
Glob (g/dl)	3.9	2.6–4.6
T. Bili (mg/dl)	1.4	0.6–2.1
AST (IU/L)	430	185–300
GGT (IU/L)	8	7–17
SDH (IU/L)	99	0–9
CK (IU/L)	8422	130–470
Na (mEq/L)	140	133–145
K (mEq/L)	3.5	2.2–4.6
CL (mEq/L)	86	100–111
TCO₂ (mEq/L)	22.6	24–34
An. gap	35	5–15

Abdominal Fluid Analysis	
Fluid color	Straw
Fluid clarity	Hazy
Supernatant color	Straw
Supernatant clarity	Clear
TP (g/dl)	1.3
NCC (/μl)	300

Cytology: There are approximately equal numbers of neutrophils and large mononuclear cells. Although the overall cellularity and protein are low, some of the neutrophils are degenerate and bacteria are seen extracellularly, predominantly rods. Some of the macrophages and neutrophils contain cytoplasmic material suggestive of bacterial remnants. There are moderate numbers of lymphocytes and rare mast cells seen. There is debris present in the background.

Interpretive Discussion

Hematology

There is a neutrophilic leukocytosis with low normal lymphocyte numbers, which most likely reflects stress, rather than inflammation. The fibrinogen is within normal limits.

Biochemical Profile

There is a mild hyperglycemia, which is consistent with stress or excitement. The marked increase in serum creatinine, and mild increase in serum phosphorus are likely the result of decreased glomerular filtration rate. A urinalysis would help differentiate causes of azotemia. The BUN concentration is at the high end of the reference range, and it is possible that in this individual, BUN could still represent a significant decrease in urea excretion if the value in health was at the low end of the reference range.

There is a slight hypocalcemia, which may be due to deposition in injured tissue.

Both serum CK and AST activities are increased, indicating muscle cell damage. The increased SDH activity also indicates some hepatocellular injury.

Serum chloride is moderately decreased. This, in combination with the decreased TCO₂, indicates an increased anion gap metabolic acidosis. Increased lactate is probably the major unmeasured anion. Lactate may have accumulated in this horse as a result of lack of perfusion to tissues, resulting in tissue hypoxia.

Abdominal Fluid Analysis

Although the quantitative indices are all within normal limits, the presence of degenerate inflammatory cells, bacteria, and debris are all consistent with an acute rupture of the intestinal tract. This would lead to third space fluid and electrolyte loss, sepsis, stress, and the laboratory abnormalities observed.

Summary

This mare experienced intestinal colic, followed by acute rupture of the involved strangulated intestine.

CASE 32

Signalment: 11-year-old intact male miniature schnauzer
History: Intermittent vomiting and diarrhea for last two weeks
Physical Examination: Tense, painful abdomen. Very fat

Hematology		Reference Range
PCV (%)	38	37–55
Hgb (g/dl)	13.2	12–18
RBC (×10⁶/µl)	5.7	5.5–8.5
MCV (fl)	67	60–72
MCHC (g/dl)	35	34–38
NCC (×10³/µl)	**17.9**	6–17
Segs (×10³/µl)	**14.2**	3–11.5
Bands (×10³/µl)	**0.5**	0–0.3
Monos (×10³/µl)	0.7	0.1–1.3
Lymphs (×10³/µl)	2.5	1–4.8
Platelets (×10³/µl)	250	200–500
TP (P) (g/dl)	**9.0**	6–8
Hemopathology: Moderate Polychromasia		

Biochemical Profile (serum was lipemic)		Reference Range
Gluc (mg/dl)	**124 (6.8)**	65–122 (3.5–6.7 mmol/L)
BUN (mg/dl)	**42 (15)**	7–28 (2.5–10.0 mmol/L)
Creat (mg/dl)	1.2	0.9–1.7
Ca (mg/dl)	9.8	9.0–11.2
Phos (mg/dl)	5.8	2.8–6.1
TP (g/dl)	**7.7**	5.4–7.4
Alb (g/dl)	3.7	2.7–4.5
Glob (g/dl)	**4.0**	1.9–3.4
T. Bili (mg/dl)	**10.8 (184.7)**	0–0.4(0–6.8 µmol/L)
Chol (mg/dl)	**1230 (32)**	130–370 (3.4–9.6 mmol/L)
ALT (IU/L)	**600**	10–120
AST (IU/L)	**540**	16–40
ALP (IU/L)	**660**	35–280
Na (mEq/L)	148	145–158
K (mEq/L)	4.3	4.1–5.5
CL (mEq/L)	110	106–127
TCO₂ (mEq/L)	24	14–27
An. gap (mEq/L)	18	8–25
Amylase (IU/L)	510	50–1250
Lipase (IU/L)	120	30–560

Urine Analysis (catheterized)			
Color	Yellow	**Urine Sediment**	
Transparency	Cloudy	WBCs/hpf	**>50**
Sp. Gr.	**1.022**	RBCs/hpf	0–1
Protein	**3+**	Epith cells/hpf	0
Gluc	Negative	Casts/lpf	0
Bilirubin	**2+**	Crystals	0
Blood	Negative	Bacteria	**Many bacilli**
pH	7.0		

Interpretive Discussion

Hematology

The PCV, hemoglobin concentration, and RBC count are at the lower end of the reference range, and it is possible that an anemia has been masked by dehydration. With a history of vomiting and diarrhea and an increased plasma protein concentration, it is possible that this animal is dehydrated. However, since the serum is lipemic, a more likely explanation for the high total plasma protein as measured by refractometry is the presence of lipids, which interfere with the reading. The presence of moderate polychromasia suggests a regenerative response. Blood loss may have caused a regenerative anemia in this dog (see summary).

Neutrophilia with a left shift indicates an inflammatory leukogram.

Biochemical Profile

The BUN concentration is only mildly increased as is the serum creatinine concentration is normal. Urine specific gravity indicates inadequate urine concentrating ability in the face of dehydration, and the BUN probably represent a renal azotemia. Since the serum creatinine concentration is normal, it is also possible that the increased BUN reflects increased urea production resulting from hemorrhage into the GI tract, followed by digestion of protein-rich blood, absorption of increased quantities of amino acids from this digested blood, and catabolism of these amino acids by the liver. The end product of this catabolism is urea, and this process results in increased BUN. However, increased plasma and serum proteins suggest that significant blood loss has not occurred.

Both plasma and serum protein concentrations are increased, but the plasma protein concentration is much higher than the serum protein concentration. Because fibrinogen is present in plasma but not in serum, one would expect the plasma protein concentration to be 0.2 to 0.4 g/dl higher than that of serum. However, the difference is often greater because plasma protein concentration is estimated using a refractometer, which measures total solids, while serum protein is measured spectrophotometrically. Increased plasma concentration of solids other than protein may falsely increase the protein estimate derived from a refractometer. The increased difference between these protein concentrations in this case is likely due to lipemia.

The hyperglobulinemia may be the result of chronic antigenic stimulation with subsequent increase in antibody production. Alternatively, the hyperglobulinemia may be the result of dehydration, but if this were the case, hyperalbuminemia would also be expected. In this case, however, it is possible the dog was hypoalbuminemic prior to the onset of dehydration and the albumin concentration increased to within the reference range after dehydration occurred. Hypoalbuminemia may have occurred secondary to chronic liver disease.

The combination of hyperbilirubinemia and increased serum ALP activity is typical of cholestasis. The increased bilirubin concentration in the urine has resulted from increased renal excretion of bilirubin and is a common result of increased serum bilirubin concentrations, especially if that bilirubin is conjugated. Although hypercholesterolemia is a nonspecific problem, cholestasis is a common cause of this abnormality and may be an explanation in this case. The magnitude of the hypercholesterolemia is unusual for cholestasis alone. Since this dog is a miniature schnauzer, and the serum is lipemic, suggesting hypertriglyceridemia and/or chylomicronemia, idiopathic hyperlipidemia is likely.

Increased serum AST and ALT activities probably resulted from hepatocyte injury. Both of these enzymes are leakage enzymes and are present in significant concentrations in hepatocytes. AST is also present in high concentrations and ALT in low concentrations in muscle, but muscle is an unlikely source of these enzymes in this case. In light of the evidence for cholestasis, hepatic origin is most likely for these enzymes in this dog.

Urinalysis

Proteinuria, pyuria and bacteruria suggest inflammation in the urinary tract. Since these are found in a voided urine sample, reproductive tract origin must also be considered. Bacteria in a voided urine sample may be contaminants but are more significant when accompanied by pyuria. Culture of this urine sample is indicated.

Summary

This dog had a suppurative cholangiohepatitis, a duodenal ulcer, and pyelonephritis. The cholangiohepatitis resulted in the cholestasis and damage to hepatocytes. The chronic antigenic stimulation caused by both cholangiohepatitis and pyelonephritis resulted in hyperglobulinemia. The mild azotemia probably resulted from pyelonephritis. The duodenal ulcer could have caused chronic blood loss, but, in light of increased protein concentrations, evidence for this is weak, and, therefore, GI tract hemorrhage is an unlikely explanation for the increased BUN.

CASE 33

Signalment: 5-year-old FS canine
History: On phenobarbital to control seizures for 2.5 years. Vomiting daily and lethargic for about 1 month.
Physical Examination: Lethargic, icteric, pendulous abdomen; arthritic and appeared older than stated age

Hematology		Reference Range
PCV (%)	40.0	37–55
Hgb (g/dl)	13.6	12–18
RBC (×10⁶/µl)	5.53	5.5–8.5
MCV (fl)	72.0	60–72
MCHC (g/dl)	34.0	34–38
NCC (×10³/µl)	**47.2**	6–17
Segs (×10³/µl)	**40.1**	3–11.5
Bands (×10³/µl)	**0.9**	0–0.3
Monos (×10³/µl)	**4.7**	0.1–1.3
Lymphs (×10³/µl)	**0.9**	1–4.8
Eos (×10³/µl)	0.5	0.1–1.2
Platelets (×10³/µl)	299	200–500
TP (P) (g/dl)	**5.5**	6–8

Hemopathology: slt toxic neutrophils, many echinocytes

Biochemical Profile		Reference Range
Gluc (mg/dl)	69	65–122
BUN (mg/dl)	**5 (1.78)**	7–28 (2.5–10.0 mmol/L)
Creat (mg/dl)	0.6	0.9–1.7
Ca (mg/dl)	**8.1 (2.02)**	9.0–11.2 (2.25–2.80 mmol/L)
Phos (mg/dl)	5.1	2.8–6.1
TP (g/dl)	**4.8**	5.4–7.4
Alb (g/dl)	**2.0**	2.7–4.5
Glob (g/dl)	2.8	1.9–3.4
T. Bili (mg/dl)	**4.5 (77)**	0–0.4 (0–6.8 µmol/L)
Chol (mg/dl)	**126 (3.28)**	130–370 (3.4–9.6 mmol/L)
ALT (IU/L)	**348**	10–120
AST (IU/L)	**176**	16–40
ALP (IU/L)	**4503**	35–280
GGT (IU/L)	**426**	0–6
Na (mEq/L)	**142**	145–158
K (mEq/L)	**3.3**	4.1–5.5
CL (mEq/L)	114	106–127
TCO₂ (mEq/L)	14.8	14–27
An. gap (mEq/L)	16.5	8–25
Lipase (IU/L)	575	30–560

Urinalysis			
Color	Orange	**Urine Sediment**	
Transparency	Cloudy	WBCs/hpf	**8–10**
Sp. Gr.	1.015	RBCs/hpf	0–2
Protein	2+	Epith cells/hpf	**80–100**
Gluc	Negative	Casts/lpf	Negative
Bilirubin	4+	Crystals	Negative
Blood	3+	Bacteria	**4+ rods**
pH	6.0		
Ketones	3+		

Coagulation Data		Reference Range
PT (seconds)	9.8	7.5–10.5
aPTT (seconds)	14.0	10.5–16.5

Interpretive Discussion

Hematology

There is a moderate neutrophilia with a mild left shift, monocytosis, and slightly toxic neutrophils were observed in the blood film. This is an inflammatory leukogram, but the lymphopenia indicates a concurrent steroid-induced component. Monocytosis is consistent with the combined leukocyte response.

Biochemical Profile

The serum glucose concentration is at the low end of the reference range and the BUN is decreased. These findings may indicate hepatic functional impairment, particularly in light of the observation of a potential stress leukogram. See discussion of serum protein below.

The serum total protein and albumin concentrations are decreased. One should consider pathologic loss of serum protein due to intestinal or renal disease, as well as blood loss. However, in this case, decreased hepatic production of albumin is yet another indication of impaired hepatocellular function.

Serum cholesterol is decreased. While one should not overinterpret decreases in some analytes, this is commonly observed in end-stage liver disease, owing to impaired hepatic lipid synthesis. This is particularly notable given the degree of hyperbilirubinemia and increases in enzyme activities indicative of cholestasis (ALP and GGT). The magnitude of increase in serum ALP activity is large enough to warrant consideration of corticosteroid induction. Likewise, the degree of increase in GGT activity may be related to steroid induction and/or hepatocellular damage, rather than cholestasis alone. The serum ALT and AST activities are moderately increased, indicating hepatocellular damage. Phenobarbital may induce increased production of several liver enzymes.

The serum sodium and potassium are decreased, and one should consider typical causes for electrolyte depletion, including pathologic losses from the gastrointestinal and urinary systems, as well as third space syndromes. Hypokalemia is a frequent observation in hepatic disease, often due to anorexia and vomiting.

Coagulation Data

The APTT and PT are normal. If hepatic disease or end-stage liver failure has progressed sufficiently, as suggested by even lower values for glucose, BUN, albumin, and cholesterol, one might expect these indices of coagulation factor synthesis to become abnormal as well.

Urinalysis

The urinary specific gravity indicates the urine is poorly concentrated and may reflect impaired concentrating ability. This may be due to the decreased BUN, since urea also plays a role in urine concentration. The concentrations of protein, ketones, bilirubin, and blood are particularly notable given this weak urine concentration. The proteinuria may be due to urinary tract inflammation/infection as indicated by the significant pyuria, bacteriuria, and presence of marked occult blood. The presence of bilirubin is not surprising given the degree of hyperbilirubinemia. The presence of ketonuria in the absence of glucosuria is unusual. Ketosis is a possible sequela to impaired oxidative lipid metabolism by the diseased liver, especially when triglyceride absorption from the GI tract or mobilization from peripheral stores is greater than hepatic functional capacity for processing.

Summary

There is prominent biochemical evidence of chronic liver failure. Phenobarbital-induced hepatopathy was also considered. Ultrasound of the liver showed an enlarged liver with numerous well-defined hypoechoic foci throughout. Masses throughout the cranial mid-abdomen had similar echogenicity as masses within liver. Cytology of a liver aspirate showed vacuolated hepatocytes, bile stasis, and a population of nonhepatic cells with a high nucleus:cytoplasm ratio, most of which were broken. Numerous cells in mitosis were observed, and neoplasia was diagnosed. Biopsy of liver revealed adenocarcinoma which effaced and replaced hepatic parenchyma, and glucocorticoid hepatopathy with severe bile stasis. The neoplasm had a neuroendocrine (potentially adrenal) pattern, and was possibly causing the steroid hepatopathy. Endocrine panel was not performed. Dog was euthanized; necropsy was not allowed.

CASE 34

Signalment: 6-year-old spayed female dog
History: Struck by car 1 month ago. Not taken to veterinarian. Dyspnea since accident. Anorexia.
Physical Examination: Emaciated and lethargic. Intestinal sounds auscultated in thorax.

Hematology		Reference Range
PCV (%)	37	37–55
Hgb (g/dl)	12.3	12–18
RBC (×10⁶/µl)	6.1	5.5–8.5
MCV (fl)	61	60–72
MCHC (g/dl)	33	34–38
NCC (×10³/µl)	16.1	6–17
Segs (×10³/µl)	**13.5**	3–11.5
Bands (×10³/µl)	0.2	0–0.3
Monos (×10³/µl)	1.0	0.1–1.3
Lymphs (×10³/µl)	**0.6**	1–4.8
Eos (×10³/µl)	0.8	0.1–1.2
Platelets (×10³/µl)	330	200–500
TP (P) (g/dl)	**3.3**	6–8
Hemopathology: Normal		

Biochemical Profile		Reference Range
Gluc (mg/dl)	77	65–122
BUN (mg/dl)	**3 (1.07)**	7–28 (2.5–10.0 mmol/L)
Creat (mg/dl)	1.5	0.9–1.7
Ca (mg/dl)	**6.3**	9.0–11.2
Phos (mg/dl)	4.4	2.8–6.1
TP (g/dl)	**2.9**	5.4–7.4
Alb (g/dl)	**0.6**	2.7–4.5
Glob (g/dl)	2.3	1.9–3.4
T. Bili (mg/dl)	**3.0 (51.3)**	0–0.4 (0–6.8 µmol/L)
Chol (mg/dl)	**102 (2.65)**	130–370 (3.4–9.6 mmol/L)
ALT (IU/L)	**170**	10–120
AST (IU/L)	**72**	16–40
ALP (IU/L)	**540**	35–280
Na (mEq/L)	146	145–158
K (mEq/L)	**6.0**	4.1–5.5
CL (mEq/L)	118	106–127
TCO₂ (mEq/L)	**11**	14–27
An. gap (mEq/L)	23	8–25
Plasma ammonia (mg/dl)	**150**	0–90

Urinalysis (catheterized)			
Color	Yellow	**Urine Sediment**	
Transparency	Clear	WBCs/hpf	0
Sp. Gr.	1.035	RBCs/hpf	0
Protein	Negative	Epith cells/hpf	0
Gluc	Negative	Casts/lpf	0
Bilirubin	1+	Crystals	**Bilirubin**
Blood	Negative	Bacteria	0
pH	5.5		

Interpretive Discussion

Hematology

This dog's erythrocyte measurements are near the lower end of their reference ranges, and there is no evidence of a regenerative response. It is possible that this dog is developing a nonregenerative anemia secondary to chronic disease. Since the MCV is at the low end of the reference range, this dog may eventually develop a microcytic (low MCV) anemia, suggesting iron deficiency.

Leukocyte abnormalities are a mature neutrophilia and lymphopenia, typical of a corticosteroid-mediated leukogram.

Biochemical Profile

Decreased BUN concentration can be caused by hepatic failure, diuresis, decreased protein intake, or treatment with anabolic steroids. BUN concentration below the reference range can also occur in normal animals. In light of other laboratory findings in this case, the decreased BUN concentration is probably due to hepatic failure and resulting failure of hepatocytes to synthesize urea. Anorexia resulting in decreased protein intake may have also contributed to this abnormality.

This dog has hypocalcemia; however, it also has severe hypoalbuminemia. In dogs with this combination of abnormalities, the measured Ca concentration should always be corrected by the formula:

Corrected Ca concentration = measured Ca concentration – albumin concentration + 3.5.

The corrected Ca concentration in this dog is 9.2 mg/dl. The serum Ca concentration, therefore, corrects into the reference range. This indicates the explanation for the hypocalcemia in this case is hypoalbuminemia. Since albumin-bound Ca is not metabolically active, this abnormality is not clinically significant.

Both plasma and serum protein concentrations are decreased. These decreases are a result of hypoalbuminemia. When interpreted in combination with other laboratory data, this abnormality is probably due to decreased albumin synthesis by the liver. Decreased protein intake can result in hypoalbuminemia and may also have played a role in this case. The albumin concentration is low enough to lead to ascites; however, ascites was not noted in this animal.

In dogs, hyperbilirubinemia can result from hemolysis, failure of hepatocyte uptake and metabolism of bilirubin, or failure to excrete bilirubin due to cholestasis or other disruption of bile flow. In this case, failure of hepatic uptake and metabolism of bilirubin is probably the major abnormality leading to hyperbilirubinemia. It is also probable the bile duct is partially blocked and cholestasis is playing a role in producing this abnormality. The increased serum ALP activity suggests cholestasis is present in this dog.

Hypocholesterolemia is probably another result of hepatic failure. The liver is a major site of cholesterol synthesis and excretion. Abnormalities of these two processes have opposite effects on serum cholesterol concentrations. In this case, synthetic failure is apparently more severe than failure to excrete cholesterol. Decreased cholesterol intake may also have contributed to the hypocholesterolemia in this dog.

Both serum ALT and AST activities are mildly increased. These enzymes leak from injured hepatocytes, and liver injury is the appropriate interpretation in this case. AST is also present in muscle cells, and muscle injury cannot be ruled out, but the mild increase of AST activity in conjunction with the increased ALT activity suggests the AST has leaked from the liver in this case.

Increased ALP activity most often results from either cholestasis or increased blood corticosteroid concentrations. In combination with other laboratory data suggesting hepatic disease, cholestasis is the most important cause of the increased ALP in this case. This dog probably had an increased blood corticosteroid concentration as suggested by the leukogram, and this may have also played a role in increasing the serum ALP activity.

Hyperkalemia may be a result of metabolic acidosis-induced shifting of K from within cells to extracellular fluid. In animals with metabolic acidosis, H ions enter cells in an attempt to equalize their concentrations in the intracellular and extracellular compartments. In order to maintain electrical neutrality, K ions must leave the cells. The net result is increased extracellular and, therefore, serum K concentrations.

The cause of the decreased total CO_2 is not certain. Since this animal has a compromised respiratory system, it is reasonable to assume that it has a respiratory acidosis. However, the total CO_2 concentration would be expected to increase in compensation for the respiratory acidosis. Since this concentration decreased rather than increased, it is reasonable to assume the dog has another abnormality causing metabolic acidosis. The normal anion gap suggests that substances such as lactate, ketones, and sulfate have not played a significant role in this acidosis. Abnormal renal regulation of acid-base balance is another possible cause of decreased total CO_2, but there is no evidence of renal dysfunction in this case.

The hyperammonemia is a result of hepatic failure. Ammonia is normally absorbed from the digestive tract and transported to the liver by the portal circulation. The liver is responsible for removing and metabolizing this ammonia. Alterations in blood flow to the liver and/or markedly decreased numbers of functional hepatocytes can result in increased blood ammonia concentrations.

Urinalysis

Bilirubinuria and the presence of bilirubin crystals are the only abnormalities in the urine. These changes reflect the increased serum bilirubin concentration. Conjugated bilirubin readily passes through glomeruli and is then excreted in the urine. The very mild increase in urine bilirubin suggests that most of the serum bilirubin is unconjugated. Interestingly, this dog is concentrating urine in the face of a very low bun.

Summary

Exploratory surgery revealed a diaphragmatic hernia through which the liver and a portion of the GI tract had passed. The liver was decreased in size and firm. Many fibrous adhesions were present. On the surgeon's recommendation, the dog was euthanized.

This dog had hepatic failure due to chronically decreased blood supply to the liver. Decreased BUN, albumin, and cholesterol concentrations suggested decreased synthetic function by the liver. Increased bilirubin and ammonia concentrations resulted from decreased delivery of these substances to the liver and, therefore, decreased removal from the blood as well as due to decreased functional hepatic mass. Cholestasis resulting from partial occlusion of the bile duct also contributed to hyperbilirubinemia. Since this was an end-stage liver disease, leakage of ALT and AST from hepatocytes was minimal due to the small number of hepatocytes remaining, and serum activities of ALT and AST were, therefore, only slightly increased.

CASE 35

Signalment: 9-month-old intact female dog
History: Struck by car 3 weeks ago. Treated for shock and released. Listless since then.
Physical Examination: Abdomen is distended and fluid-filled.

Hematology		Reference Range
PCV (%)	**30**	37–55
Hgb (g/dl)	**10.3**	12–18
RBC (×10⁶/µl)	**5.45**	5.5–8.5
MCV (fl)	**55**	60–72
MCHC (g/dl)	34	34–38
Retics (/µl)	42	<60
NCC (×10³/µl)	16	6–17
Segs (×10³/µl)	**12.8**	3–11.5
Bands (×10³/µl)	**0.5**	0–0.3
Lymphs (×10³/µl)	2.7	1–4.8
Platelets (×10³/µl)	270	200–500
TP (P) (g/dl)	6.5	6–8

Hemopathology: Slight hypochromasia, moderate number of keratocytes

Biochemical Profile		Reference Range
Gluc (mg/dl)	65	65–122
BUN (mg/dl)	25	7–28
Creat (mg/dl)	1.2	0.9–1.7
Ca (mg/dl)	**8.4 (2.1)**	9.0–11.2 (2.25–2.80 mmol/L)
Phos (mg/dl)	6.0	2.8–6.1
TP (g/dl)	5.8	5.4–7.4
Alb (g/dl)	**2.5**	2.7–4.5
Glob (g/dl)	3.3	1.9–3.4
T. Bili	**0.5 (8.5)**	0–0.4 (0–6.8 µmol/L)
Chol (mg/dl)	170	130–370
ALT (IU/L)	23	10–120
AST (IU/L)	28	16–40
ALP (IU/L)	51	35–280
Na (mEq/L)	**139**	145–158
K (mEq/L)	5.2	4.1–5.5
CL (mEq/L)	**105**	106–127
TCO₂ (mEq/L)	15	14–27
An. gap (mEq/L)	24	8–25

Urinalysis (voided)			
Color	Dark yellow	**Urine Sediment**	
Transparency	Clear	WBCs/hpf	0
Sp. Gr.	1.030	RBCs/hpf	0
Protein	Negative	Epith cells/hpf	0
Gluc	Negative	Casts/lpf	0
Bilirubin	**3+**	Crystals	**Bilirubin**
Blood	Negative	Bacteria	0
pH	6.0		

Body Fluid Analysis			
Color	Red-brown	**Differential**	
Transparency	Hazy	Neutrophils	74%
TP (g/dl)	3.8	Lymphs	5%
NCC (/µl)	8800	Macrophages	21%

Other observations: Neutrophils are nondegenerate. Lymphocytes are uniformly small. Large mononuclear cells are a mixture of reactive mesothelial cells and macrophages. Macrophages contain large amounts of blue-green pigment, suggestive of bile. No micro-organisms are evident. Moderate numbers of erythrocytes are present.

Interpretive Discussion

Hematology

This dog has a nonregenerative anemia. The indices reveal that this anemia is microcytic and borderline hypochromic. These abnormalities, in combination with the presence of hypochromia and keratocytes observed on the blood film, indicate iron deficiency. Serum iron concentration should be measured in this dog. Although the most common cause of iron deficiency is chronic blood loss, there is no history of such blood loss in this case. In most such cases, examination of feces will reveal the presence of blood. GI parasites such as hookworms, should also be considered.

Borderline neutrophilia with a slight left shift suggests a mild tissue demand for neutrophils, and, therefore, a mild inflammatory process. It is likely that the anemia is non-regenerative due to the presence of inflammation (anemia of inflammatory disease).

Biochemical Profile

The blood glucose concentration is at the bottom of the reference range. Decreased carbohydrate intake or decreased hepatic production are possible causes. Since there is little evidence of hepatic failure in this case, decreased intake appears to be the most likely explanation. Alternatively, it may be normal for this dog.

The hypocalcemia is a result of hypoalbuminemia. In dogs with both hypocalcemia and hypoalbuminemia, a corrected serum Ca concentration should be calculated by the formula:

Corrected Ca concentration = measured Ca concentration – albumin concentration + 3.5.

The corrected Ca concentration in this dog is 9.4 mg/dl. The serum Ca concentration, therefore, corrects into the reference range. Since albumin-bound Ca is not metabolically active, this abnormality is not clinically significant.

The mild hypoalbuminemia is probably due to decreased protein intake or decreased amino acid absorption from the GI tract. Evidence of hepatic failure is not present, and urine protein concentration is normal; therefore, decreased albumin production by the liver and increased albumin loss through the kidneys are unlikely. In light of the anemia and the evidence of iron deficiency, chronic blood loss should be considered as a cause of hypoalbuminemia in this case; however, globulin concentration usually decreases proportionally with albumin concentration during blood loss. The globulin concentration may, however, have been increased in this dog due to chronic antigenic stimulation, and this would explain a normal globulin concentration despite blood loss severe enough to result in hypoalbuminemia.

The combination of increased serum and urine bilirubin concentrations suggests disruption in the hepatic excretion of conjugated bilirubin. The serum bilirubin concentration, while increased, appears inappropriately low in light of the marked increase in urine bilirubin concentration. Dogs have a low renal threshold for bilirubin, and, in dogs with abnormalities of hepatic conjugated bilirubin excretion, urine bilirubin concentration may increase prior to increases in serum bilirubin concentration, or urine bilirubin concentration may be markedly increased while serum bilirubin concentration is only mildly increased.

Hyponatremia and hypochloremia were probably caused by dilution of these electrolytes in an increased volume of extracellular fluid. This increased fluid volume is a result of accumulation of fluid in the peritoneal cavity. This "third-spacing" phenomenon commonly results in hyponatremia and hypochloremia.

Urinalysis

Marked bilirubinuria and presence of bilirubin crystals are the only abnormalities in the urinalysis. These changes probably resulted from increased passage of conjugated bilirubin into the blood with subsequent renal excretion. Either cholestasis or rupture of the bile duct or gall bladder could be an underlying cause.

Abdominal Fluid Analysis

Based on the total nucleated cell count and on the predominance of neutrophils, the peritoneal fluid should be classified as an exudate. Since neutrophils are nondegenerate and bacteria are absent, this is probably a nonseptic exudate. The pigment noted in macrophages is suggestive of bile and, therefore, gall bladder or bile duct rupture are likely.

Summary

Exploratory surgery revealed a ruptured gall bladder. Due to severe adhesions throughout the peritoneal cavity, the owner was offered a guarded prognosis. The owner opted for euthanasia.

Bilirubin leaking with bile into this dog's peritoneal cavity was reabsorbed through the peritoneal wall. The bilirubin entered the blood and was efficiently excreted by the kidneys. As a result, serum bilirubin concentration increased only slightly while urine bilirubin concentration increased markedly. Serum activities of the hepatic leakage enzymes, ALT and AST, did not increase since there was no direct liver injury. Serum activity of ALP did not increase since there was no cholestasis.

CASE 36

Signalment: 2-year-old male mixed breed dog
History: Weight loss, lethargy
Physical Examination: Thin dog, pendulous abdomen
Hematology: Unremarkable

Biochemical Profile		Reference Range
Gluc (mg/dl)	**64 (3.5)**	65–122 (3.5–6.7 mmol/L)
BUN (mg/dl)	**6 (2.1)**	7–28 (2.5–10.0 mmol/L)
Creat (mg/dl)	1.0	0.9–1.7
Ca (mg/dl)	**7.4 (1.85)**	9.0–11.2 (2.25–2.80 mmol/L)
Phos (mg/dl)	2.8	2.8–6.1
TP (g/dl)	**4.2**	5.4–7.4
Alb (g/dl)	**1.2**	2.7–4.5
Glob (g/dl)	3.0	1.9–3.4
T. Bili (mg/dl)	0.4	0–0.4
Chol (mg/dl)	**65 (1.7)**	130–370 (3.4–9.6 mmol/L)
ALT (IU)	**30**	10–120
ALP (IU)	260	35–280
Bile Acids (μmol/L)	**30**	3.0–9.0
Na (mEq/L)	146	145–158
K (mEq/L)	4.1	4.1–5.5
CL (mEq/L)	115	106–127

Abdominal Fluid Analysis	
TP (g/dl)	1.0
NCC (/μl)	1500
Segs (%)	60
Lymphs (%)	22
Macrophages (%)	18
Morphology: neutrophils nondegenerate	

Interpretive Discussion

Biochemical Profile

A number of factors in the profile suggest liver failure. These include a borderline low glucose, low BUN, hypoproteinemia characterized by severe hypoalbuminemia, and a markedly low cholesterol concentration. Hepatic enzymes are often normal with end stage liver disease. An alternative, but less likely, possibility for this pattern is severe starvation. The increased bile acids indicate decreased liver function and help confirm end stage liver disease.

Hypocalcemia corrects to normal, given the hypoalbuminemia.

Body Fluid Analysis

The abdominal fluid has the typical features of a transudate. With end-stage liver disease this is due to a combination of hypoalbuminemia and increased portal blood pressure resulting in transudation of fluid into the cavity.

Summary

Hepatic cirrhosis; end-stage liver disease.

CASE 37

Signalment: 3-month-old intact female dog
History: Anorexia, depression, and diarrhea of one week duration. Poor growth rate.
Physical Examination: Severe, diffuse dermatitis with multifocal ulcerative lesions.

Hematology		Reference Range
PCV (%)	**13**	37–55
Hgb (g/dl)	**4.5**	12–18
RBC (×10⁶/μl)	**2.5**	5.5–8.5
MCV (fl)	**52**	60–72
MCHC (g/dl)	35	34–38
Retics (/μl)	**2.5**	<60
NCC (×10³/μl)	**1.6**	6–17
Segs (×10³/μl)	**0.5**	3–11.5
Bands (×10³/μl)	0.1	0–0.3
Monos (×10³/μl)	0.1	0.1–1.3
Lymphs (×10³/μl)	**0.9**	1–4.8
Platelets (×10³/μl)	340	200–500
TP (P) (g/dl)	**3.4**	6–8

Hemopathology: Markedly toxic neutrophils, few RBC fragments

Biochemical Profile		Reference Range
Gluc (mg/dl)	**40 (2.2)**	65–122 (3.5–6.7 mmol/L)
BUN (mg/dl)	**4 (1.43)**	7–28 (2.5–10.0 mmol/L)
Creat (mg/dl)	0.3	0.9–1.7
Ca (mg/dl)	**7.8 (1.95)**	9.0–11.2 (2.25–2.80 mmol/L)
Phos (mg/dl)	**2.0 (0.65)**	2.8–6.1 (0.9–2.0 mmol/L)
TP (g/dl)	**2.9**	5.4–7.4
Alb (g/dl)	**1.7**	2.7–4.5
Glob (g/dl)	**1.2**	1.9–3.4
T. Bili (mg/dl)	0.2	0–0.4
Chol (mg/dl)	142	130–370
ALT (IU/L)	15	10–120
AST (IU/L)	22	16–40
ALP (IU/L)	63	35–280
GGT (IU/L)	6	0–6
Na (mEq/L)	**141**	145–158
K (mEq/L)	**3.7**	4.1–5.5
CL (mEq/L)	114	106–127
TCO₂ (mEq/L)	17	14–27
An. gap (mEq/L)	14	8–25
Fasting Bile acids (μmol/L)	**88**	<10
Iron (μg/dl)	**50 (8.95)**	60–110 (10.7–19.7 μmol/L)

Urinalysis (cystocentesis)			
Color	Yellow	**Urine Sediment**	
Transparency	Clear	WBCs/hpf	0–2
Sp. Gr.	1.029	RBCs/hpf	0
Protein	Negative	Epith cells/hpf	0
Gluc	2+	Casts/lpf	0
Bilirubin	Negative	Crystals	0
Blood	Negative	Bacteria	0
pH	5.0		

Interpretive Discussion

Hematology

This dog has a severe nonregenerative anemia. The anemia in this dog is microcytic, and the serum iron concentration is decreased, suggesting iron deficiency secondary to chronic blood loss. Alternately, microcytic anemia is also seen in dogs with portocaval syndrome, in which case, serum iron may or may not be decreased, and anemia may be secondary to other abnormalities in iron metabolism. Red blood cell fragmentation is a typical finding in iron deficiency anemia. While iron deficiency anemia is often regenerative, this dog's bone marrow may not be adequately responding, perhaps due to viral damage or concurrent anemia of chronic disease.

Severe leukopenia has resulted from a combination of neutropenia and lymphopenia. In a young dog with diarrhea as well as neutropenia and lymphopenia, parvovirus infection with virus-induced bone marrow damage should be a strong consideration. Acute bacterial enteritis resulting in endotoxemia may result in a similar leukogram. The presence of toxic neutrophils suggests that the bone marrow is rapidly producing neutrophils, and this may signal early recovery of previously suppressed neutrophil production, or may be a response to loss of neutrophils due to rapid destruction or emigration into tissues as would occur with endotoxemia or overwhelming tissue demand for neutrophils, respectively.

Platelets are adequate, indicating chronic marrow failure is not present.

Biochemical Profile

Hypoglycemia probably resulted from decreased hepatic glucose production. Numerous diseases can result in hypoglycemia, but, in light of other laboratory data, hepatic failure is the most likely cause of hypoglycemia in this dog. The decreased blood supply to the liver which occurs with portosystemic shunts can result in liver atrophy. Such a liver cannot play its normal role in maintenance of blood glucose concentrations. A second possibility, in light of the decreased neutrophil concentration, is that the dog has bacteremia or endotoxemia which may result in hypoglycemia. A third possibility is that glucose is being lost through the urinary tract (see discussion of glucosuria).

Both the BUN and serum creatinine concentrations are decreased. Since there is evidence of hepatic failure, it is possible that the decreased BUN concentration resulted from decreased liver production of urea. However, the concurrent decrease in serum creatinine concentration suggests that increased renal clearance of both urea and creatinine has occurred. This dog has a glucosuria, and this may have caused osmotic diuresis. With chronic diuresis, increased renal excretion of both urea and creatinine and, subsequently, decreased BUN and serum creatinine concentrations can result.

This dog has both hypocalcemia and hypoalbuminemia, and a corrected serum Ca concentration should, therefore, be calculated by the formula:

Corrected Ca concentration = measured Ca concentration – albumin concentration + 3.5.

The corrected Ca concentration in this dog is 9.6 mg/dl. The serum Ca concentration, therefore, corrects into the normal range. Since albumin-bound Ca is not metabolically active, the hypocalcemia is not clinically significant.

Hypophosphatemia occurs most commonly in hypercalcemic disorders such as primary hyperparathyroidism and pseudohyperparathyroidism, but these are unlikely in a 3-month-old dog. Other causes include dietary phosphate or vitamin D deficiency, malabsorption syndrome, diabetes mellitus, and canine Fanconi-like syndrome. This dog appears to have a renal tubular defect (see discussion of glucosuria), and it is possible that this defect is part of a canine Fanconi-like syndrome. In such a syndrome, inadequate tubular reabsorption of phosphate results in excessive loss of phosphate in the urine.

The hypoproteinemia is the result of both hypoalbuminemia and hypoglobulinemia. These abnormalities, in combination with anemia, indicate that blood loss should be considered. In this case, it is likely chronic liver disease is also contributing to hypoalbuminemia.

This dog's serum bilirubin concentration, serum alkaline phosphatase (ALP) activity, and gamma glutamyl transferase (GGT) activity are normal, suggesting that cholestasis is not occurring. While most forms of liver failure result in some degree of cholestasis, liver failure resulting from a portosystemic shunt usually does not. These normal values, in combination with the history and other laboratory abnormalities, suggest that a portosystemic shunt is likely. Since this is a young dog, a slight increase in ALP of bone origin would not have been unusual. Despite evidence of hepatic disease, serum ALT and AST activities are normal. Serum activities of hepatic leakage enzymes such as ALT and AST may be normal to increased in dogs with portosystemic shunts.

The hyponatremia and hypokalemia may have resulted from diuresis induced by glucosuria. It is also possible this dog's tubular function defect includes abnormal reabsorption of Na and K.

Markedly increased fasting bile acid concentration can result from decreased hepatic blood flow, hepatic failure, or cholestasis. In this case, decreased hepatic blood flow and subsequent hepatic failure are the most likely explanations.

Blood loss is the most common cause of decreased serum iron concentration in animals, although nursing animals have low serum iron due to inadequate dietary intake. In this case, however, the decreased serum iron concentration is probably due to the presence of a portosystemic shunt. The cause of the decreased serum iron concentration in dogs with portosystemic shunts is not known, but appears to be related to iron sequestration in tissues such as liver and/or defects in the transport of iron. Some cases also have intermittent gastrointestinal bleeding associated with pica.

Urinalysis

Moderate glucosuria in an animal with a low or normal blood glucose suggests a lowered renal threshold for glucose and, therefore, a renal tubular absorption defect. Such a defect may be confined to glucose absorption only, or may include defective absorption of several substances. As previously noted, this dog may also have defective absorption of phosphate, sodium, and potassium. If this is the case, this is probably a form of canine Fanconi-like syndrome. Measurement of the fractional excretion of phosphate, sodium, and potassium would have helped in assessing this possibility.

Summary

This dog had a portosystemic shunt. Hypoglycemia, decreased BUN concentration, hypoalbuminemia, and increased serum bile acid concentrations probably resulted from decreased hepatic blood flow and subsequent hepatic failure. Microcytosis has been reported as common in dogs with portosystemic shunts and is frequently related to low serum iron concentrations. This dog also has a renal tubular defect. Glucosuria in the presence of hypoglycemia, hypophosphatemia, hyponatremia, and hypokalemia are probably a result of defective tubular reabsorption of these substances. This defect is probably a canine Fanconi-like syndrome. Neutropenia does not typically occur in either portosystemic shunts or canine Fanconi-like syndrome, and this dog may have a concurrent enteric infection, most likely caused by parvovirus or endotoxin-producing bacteria, resulting in this abnormality.

CASE 38

Signalment: 6-month-old intact male dog
History: Struck by a car on Day 1

Physical Examination: Pale mucous membranes. Day 1 blood sample obtained 12 hours after accident.

Hematology	Day 1	Day 6	Reference Range
PCV (%)	29	35	37–55
Hgb (g/dl)	9.6	11.5	12–18
RBC (×10⁶/µl)	4.7	5.1	5.5–8.5
MCV (fl)	62	69	60–72
MCHC (g/dl)	33	33	34–38
Retics (/µl)	47	304	<60
NCC (×10³/µl)	22.7	20.0	6–17
Segs (×10³/µl)	22.0	12.0	3–11.5
Bands (×10³/µl)	0	2.0	0–0.3
Monos (×10³/µl)	0	1.0	0.1–1.3
Lymphs (×10³/µl)	0.7	5.0	1–4.8
Platelets (×10³/µl)	340	460	150–900
TP (P) (g/dl)	5.4	6.5	6–8

Hemopathology: No abnormalities on Day 1. Moderate anisocytosis and polychromasia on Day 6,

Biochemical Profile	Day 1	Day 6	Reference Range
Gluc (mg/dl)	125 (6.9)	105	65–122 (3.5–6.7 mmol/L)
BUN (mg/dl)	9	13	7–28
Creat (mg/dl)	1.1	1.3	0.9–1.7
Ca (mg/dl)	8.9 (2.22)	9.3	9.0–11.2 (2.25–2.80 mmol/L)
Phos (mg/dl)	5.5	5.6	2.8–6.1
TP (g/dl)	5.0	6.0	5.4–7.4
Alb (g/dl)	3.4	4.0	2.7–4.5
Glob (g/dl)	1.6	2.0	1.9–3.4
T. Bili (mg/dl)	0.3	0.4	0–0.4
Chol (mg/dl)	210	180	130–370
ALT (IU/L)	1098	150	10–120
AST (IU/L)	948	80	16–40
ALP (IU/L)	302	295	35–280
Na (mEq/L)	150	147	145–158
K (mEq/L)	4.8	4.7	4.1–5.5
CL (mEq/L)	120	121	106–127
TCO₂ (mEq/L)	12	21	14–27
An. gap (mEq/L)	23	10	8–25

Urinalysis (catheterized)—obtained on Day 1			
Color	Yellow	**Urine Sediment**	
Transparency	Clear	WBCs/hpf	1–2
Sp. Gr.	1.019	RBCs/hpf	3–5
Protein	Trace	Epith cells/hpf	0
Gluc	Negative	Casts/lpf	0
Bilirubin	Negative	Crystals	0
Blood	Negative	Bacteria	0
pH	6.5		

Interpretive Discussion

Hematology

This dog is anemic on both days. The anemia is more severe on Day 1 and is nonregenerative. Since the Day 1 blood sample was obtained 12 hours after the accident, it is likely that the anemia is due to acute blood loss. The concurrent hypoproteinemia (see discussion below) also supports blood loss as the cause of this anemia. Increased polychromasia and reticulocyte count are not evident in blood until 2 to 4 days following acute blood loss. While the anemia appears nonregenerative on the initial sample, by Day 6, the erythrocyte values have increased, and there is evidence of increased erythrocyte production (increased polychromasia and reticulocyte count). This dog is, therefore, responding appropriately to the blood loss.

The MCHC is slightly decreased on both days. This value should not have been affected by the blood loss on Day 1, and may, therefore, be normal for this dog. Although normal on both days, the MCV increased between Day 1 and Day 6, probably due to increased erythrocyte production resulting in increased number of large, immature erythrocytes.

The dog has a mature neutrophilia and lymphopenia on Day 1. This is compatible with a corticosteroid-mediated leukogram, resulting from stress associated with pain or trauma.

Neutrophilia and a left shift on Day 6 are typical of an inflammatory leukogram. Tissue injury associated with the accident probably incited an inflammatory response. An infectious etiology cannot be eliminated, however.

Biochemical Profile

Mild hyperglycemia on Day 1 resulted from stress. The presence of a stress leukogram supports this explanation.

Slight hypocalcemia may be normal in this dog since young animals commonly have slightly lower serum Ca concentrations than adults. However, the serum Ca concentration returned to within the reference range on Day 6, suggesting that this is the more normal value for this dog. It is possible that the hypocalcemia on Day 1 resulted from loss of albumin and albumin-bound Ca during hemorrhage.

Hypoproteinemia and hypoglobulinemia on Day 1 probably resulted from loss of protein during hemorrhage. Although the serum albumin concentration is in the normal range, this might actually be low for this animal. The serum albumin concentration increased by Day 6, implying that this is the more normal concentration for this dog. All protein concentrations returned to within the reference ranges by Day 6, indicating that compensatory mechanisms had replaced the protein lost through hemorrhage.

Both serum ALT and AST activities are markedly increased on Day 1, but decrease to nearly normal by Day 6. These increases suggest liver and/or muscle injury. High concentrations of ALT are present in the liver and lower concentrations are present in muscle. The marked increase in ALT in this case, therefore, probably resulted from liver injury, but muscle injury may have also contributed. Aspartate aminotransferase (AST) is present in high concentrations in both liver and muscle, and both tissues may be sources of AST in this case. Liver and muscle trauma may explain these increased enzyme activities on Day 1. Shock with subsequent hypoxia and tissue injury can also result in leakage and increased serum activities of both enzymes. Regardless of the underlying cause of their leakage, the decreasing activities of both enzymes by Day 6 imply the damage was acute, and it is no longer active.

Increased alkaline phosphatase (ALP) activities may be normal for this dog. Young, growing animals commonly have slightly to moderately increased serum ALP activity since, due to active bone growth, increased amounts of ALP are released from osteoblasts.

There is a slight decrease in the total CO_2 on Day 1, suggesting metabolic acidosis. Hypovolemic shock leading to tissue hypoxia may have resulted in production of acid metabolites, and decreased renal blood flow may have interfered with renal acid-base regulation. The anion gap, while still within the reference range, is higher on Day 1 as compared to Day 6, and this may have resulted from increased blood concentrations of anions such as lactate.

Urinalysis

In light of the relatively dilute urine (specific gravity = 1.019), the urine concentration of erythrocytes may be slightly increased. Mild hematuria may have resulted from trauma.

Summary

This dog had a dislocated hip and broken femur. Surgery was performed between Days 1 and 6. The dog's recovery was uneventful. This case demonstrates a normal response to acute blood loss. It also demonstrates the importance of serial measurement of serum enzyme activities in animals with increases of these activities. Steady or increasing activities of these enzymes indicates active and continuing damage to the tissue(s) of origin. Decreasing activities usually indicate that the injury has ceased and/or is resolving.

CASE 39

Signalment: 5-year-old cocker spaniel

History: Presented for anorexia and dark orange urine and feces. Dog had ITP 2 years previously, and has been given phenobarbital (100 mg bid) for epilepsy for several years.

Hematology		Reference Range
PCV (%)	13	37–55
RBC (×10⁶/µl)	1.95	5.5–8.5
Hgb (g/dl)	4.6	12–18
MCV (fl)	67	60–72
MCHC (g/dl)	35	34–38
Retics (/µl)	0	0–60,000
NCC (×10³/µl)	54.9	6.0–17.0
Metas (×10³/µl)	1.1	0
Bands (×10³/µl)	6.0	0–0.3
Segs (×10³/µl)	43.4	3.0–11.5
Lymphs (×10³/µl)	1.1	1.0–4.8
Monos (×10³/µl)	2.2	0.2–1.4
Eos (×10³/µl)	0.5	0.1–1.2
NRBCs (×10³/µl)	0.5	0
Platelets (×10³/µl)	260	200–500
TP (P) (g/dl)	6.3	6.0–8.0

Hemopathology: occasional imperfect spheres, some slight agglutination

Coombs test: **positive**

Bone marrow aspirate
Megakaryocytes present. Myeloid and erythroid hyperplasia, with normal maturation up to metarubricyte stage. M:E ratio decreased slightly. Rare erythrophagocytosis

Biochemical Profile		Reference Range
Gluc (mg/dl)	56 (3.1)	65–122 (3.5–6.7 mmol/L)
BUN (mg/dl)	56 (19.9)	7–28 (2.5–10 mmol/L)
Creat (mg/dl)	0.6	0.6–1.5
Ca (mg/dl)	8.5 (2.1)	9.0–11.2 (2.25–2.80 mmol/L)
Phos (mg/dl)	6.4 (2.1)	2.8–6.1 (0.9–2.0 mmol/L)
TP (g/dl)	3.8	5.4–7.4
Alb (g/dl)	1.5	2.7–4.5
Glob (g/dl)	2.3	1.9–3.4
T. Bili (mg/dl)	35.8 (612.2)	0–0.4 (0–6.84 µmol/L)
Chol (mg/dl)	64 (1.6)	130–370 (3.4–9.6 mmol/L)
ALT (IU)	70	16–40
ALP (IU)	566	18–141
GGT (IU)	15	0–6
Na (mEq/L)	157	145–158
K (mEq/L)	3.2	4.1–5.5
CL (mEq/L)	135	106–127
TCO₂ (mEq/L)	9.5	14–27
An. gap (mEq/L)	16	8–26

Urinalysis	
Color	brown
Transparency	cloudy
Sp. Gr.	1.022
Bilirubin	++++
No other abnormal findings	

Interpretive Discussion

Hematology

The dog is markedly anemic. Reticulocytes are not increased, indicating that the anemia is not regenerative. The presence of the imperfect spherocytes and agglutination is suggestive of immune mediated hemolytic anemia, possibly very acute, or with destruction of precursors. An unexplained nonregenerative anemia, when platelets and neutrophils are normal and increased, respectively, triggered a bone marrow aspirate. The bone marrow aspirate findings further substantiated immune mediated hemolytic anemia with destruction of polychromatophilic cells.

Neutrophilia, increased immature neutrophils, and monocytosis are indicative of inflammation.

If the animal has not received a previous transfusion, a positive Coombs' test is suggestive of immune mediated hemolytic anemia.

Bone Marrow

In light of marked erythroid response in marrow, anemia is either very acute, and will respond, or precursors are being destroyed. Because imperfect spherocytes are present on blood film, the latter is more likely.

Biochemical Profile

The serum glucose concentration is decreased. Differentials should include insulinoma and, in this patient, end stage liver disease, since the animal is also hypoalbuminemic and hypocholesterolemic.

The BUN is increased, and although the creatinine is within the reference range, one would expect the animal to be concentrating greater than 1.022 if the azotemia is prerenal. One should consider if the animal is bleeding into the GI tract, increasing the BUN, or since IMHA is suspected based on the hematology, if the animal has hemolysis with subsequent hemoglobinuric nephrosis. If the animal does have end-stage liver disease, one would expect the BUN to be decreased as well, so the increase in BUN is slightly confusing. The mild increase in serum phosphorus suggests decreased glomerular filtration rate.

The serum calcium is decreased due to hypoalbuminemia.

The serum total protein concentration is decreased due to hypoalbuminemia. Since the globulin is within the reference range, liver failure would be the best differential, since the animal is not proteinuric. Another consideration would be that blood loss is causing the anemia and hypoproteinemia, but there is no clinical evidence of blood loss.

The serum bilirubin concentration is markedly increased and may be due to hemolysis, liver failure, or cholestasis or some combination of the three. The ALT is only slightly increased, indicating mild hepatocellular damage. The ALP activity is increased, as is GGT activity, indicating cholestasis. Alternatively, enzymes may be induced by phenobarbital.

Serum total CO_2 is decreased, suggesting metabolic acidosis. This may be secondary to lactic acidosis associated with marked anemia. Increased sodium and chloride suggest hypertonic dehydration or administration of hypertonic fluid. The hypokalemia in conjunction with metabolic acidosis (which sould have caused an increased potassium) suggests a whole body potassium effect.

Urinalysis

The marked bilirubinuria reflects conjugated hyperbilirubinemia. Specific gravity is discussed above.

Summary

Immune mediated hemolytic anemia; liver failure, renal dysfunction. The dog died, and necropsy showed severe chronic micronodular cirrhosis and cholestasis, possibly related to phenobarbital. Bone marrow showed myeloid and erythroid hyperplasia. Examination of the kidneys revealed severe hemoglobinemic nephrosis with mild chronic interstitial nephritis.

CASE 40

Signalment: 8-month-old German shepherd
History: Lethargic, "poor doer," weight loss

Hematology		Reference Range
PCV (%)	34	37–55
MCV (fl)	52	60–72
NCC (×10³/μl)	44.6	6–17
Segs (×10³/μl)	38.0	3–11.5
Bands (×10³/μl)	2.2	0–0.3
Lymphs (×10³/μl)	3.1	1.0–4.8
Monos (×10³/μl)	0.9	0.2–1.4
Eos (×10³/μl)	0.4	0.1–1.2
Platelets (×10³/μl)	Adequate	200–500

Biochemical Profile		Reference Range
Gluc (mg/dl)	87	65–122
BUN (mg/dl)	6 (2.1)	7–28 (2.5–10.0 mmol/L)
Creat (mg/dl)	0.5	0.9–1.7
Ca (mg/dl)	8.6 (2.15)	9.0–11.2 (2.25–2.80 mmol/L)
Phos (mg/dl)	5.6	2.8–6.1
TP (g/dl)	4.3	5.4–7.4
Alb (g/dl)	2.4	2.7–4.5
Glob (g/dl)	1.9	1.9–3.4
T. Bili (mg/dl)	0.4	0–0.4
Chol (mg/dl)	75 (1.95)	130–370 (3.4–9.6 mmol/L)
ALT (IU)	250	10–120
ALP (IU)	129	35–280
GGT (IU)	7	0–6
Na (mEq/L)	154	145–158
K (mEq/L)	4.1	4.1–5.5
CL (mEq/L)	126	106–127
TCO₂ (mEq/L)	22.3	14–27
An. gap (mEq/L)	10	8–26
Bile acids (mmol/L) (pre)	88.5	<10
Serum iron (μg/dl)	22	60–100

Interpretive Discussion

Hematology

The dog has mild anemia that is not characterized by a reticulocyte count. The anemia is microcytic suggesting iron deficiency. Microcytosis should also prompt consideration of a portosystemic shunt in a young dog. The marked hypoferremia suggests iron deficiency is the cause of the microcytosis. There is a marked leukocytosis characterized by neutrophilia with a left shift; this is interpreted as an inflammatory leukogram.

Biochemical Profile

The decreased BUN suggests reduced biosynthesis of urea by the liver. The same may be interpreted for cholesterol and albumin. There is a moderate increase in ALT suggesting a mild degree of hepatocellular injury. The prominently increased bile acid concentration confirms a defect in hepatic function. The bilirubin and ALP do not indicate cholestasis. The slight increase in GGT is of questionable significance.

Hypocalcemia corrects to normal when the hypoalbuminemia is considered.

Summary

The findings of reduced hepatic biosynthesis with retention of bile acids in a young dog are highly suggestive of portosystemic shunt.

CASE 41

Signalment: 8-year-old male Samoyed
History: Diarrhea
Physical Examination: Recumbent, arrested prior to treatment

Hematology		Reference Range
PCV (%)	18	37–55
Retics (/µl)	197,830 (7.3%)	<60,000
MCV (fl)	66	60–72
NCC (×10³/µl)	78.0	6–17
Segs (×10³/µl)	44.5	3–11.5
Bands (×10³/µl)	14.8	0–0.3
Metas (×10³/µl)	3.9	0
Myelocytes (×10³/µl)	0.8	0
Monos (×10³/µl)	0.8	0.1–1.3
Lymphs (×10³/µl)	3.1	1–4.8
NRBC (×10³/µl)	9.4	0
Platelets (×10³/µl)	158	200–500

Hemopathology: Increased polychromasia, target cells, giant platelets, toxic neutrophils.

Biochemical Profile		Reference Range
Gluc (mg/dl)	580 (31.9)	65–122 (3.5–6.7 mmol/L)
BUN (mg/dl)	98 (35)	7–28 (2.5–10.0 mmol/L)
Creat (mg/dl)	3.1 (274)	0.9–1.7 (80–150 µmol/L)
Ca (mg/dl)	9.6	9.0–11.2
Phos (mg/dl)	13.1 (4.2)	2.8–6.1 (0.9–2.0 mmol/L)
TP (g/dl)	4.7	5.4–7.4
Alb (g/dl)	2.4	2.7–4.5
T. Bili (mg/dl)	0.6 (10.3)	0–0.4 (0–6.8 µmol/L)
Chol (mg/dl)	246	130–370
ALT (IU)	1031	10–120
ALP (IU)	2500	35–280
Na (mEq/L)	130	145–158
K (mEq/L)	6.5	4.1–5.5
CL (mEq/L)	87	106–127
TCO₂ (mEq/L)	10.6	14–27
An. gap (mEq/L)	39	8–26

Urinalysis	
Sp. Gr.	1.017
Gluc	2+
Protein	0
Ketones	0
No other abnormalities present	

Interpretive Discussion

Hematology

There is moderate regenerative anemia. Considering the hypoproteinemia, hemorrhage is the most likely cause. The nucleated RBC are interpreted as part of the regenerative response. There is a marked leukocytosis characterized by prominent neutrophilia and a left shift to myelocytes indicating inflammation.

Biochemical Profile and Urinalysis

There is marked hyperglycemia. This is associated with an expected glucosuria. The magnitude of hyperglycemia should prompt consideration of diabetes. The lack of urine ketones makes the diagnosis more difficult.

Moderate azotemia is indicated by increased concentrations of BUN and creatinine. The specific gravity indicates minimal concentrating ability in the face of azotemia. This suggests an element of primary renal disease. Alternatively, medullary wash out (see low sodium) may be contributing to the decreased concentrating ability. The increased phosphorus is compatible with decreased glomerular filtration.

The hypoproteinemia along with regenerative anemia is compatible with blood loss.

There is a marked increase in ALT activity indicating hepatocellular injury. Diabetes is associated with fat mobilization to the liver; this may result in modest ALT activities. The magnitude of this ALT suggests more severe injury. There is also an element of cholestasis indicated by the marked increase in ALP and a minimal increase in bilirubin.

The hyponatremia is likely due to urinary sodium loss secondary to glucosuria (osmotic diuresis). Additionally, cellular water may move from the intracellular compartment into the ions extracellular fluid compartment, diluting serum sodium (1.6 mEq/L decrease in sodium for every 100 mg/dl increase in glucose). The hyperkalemia is probably due to a shift of potassium ions out of cells in exchange for hydrogen ions, which enter cells during metabolic acidosis. Another possibility is that the animal is becoming oliguric and retaining potassium.

Increased anion gap is due to the presence of "unmeasured" anions. In this dog, these likely include phosphates, as well as lactate, since the dog is markedly anemic. In addition, because this dog is diabetic, ketones may be unmeasured anions. Although this dog does not have ketonuria, hydroxybutylic acid is not detected by routine tests for ketonuria, and therefore may be present.

Summary

Further evaluation led to the findings of diabetes mellitus and hepatic lipidosis. The enlarged, fragile liver had led to a fractured liver. This latter injury likely contributed to the magnitude of the ALT increase.

CASE 42

Signalment: 4-year-old DSH cat
History: Anorexia, weight loss, depression
Physical Examination: Thin, icteric mucous membranes

Hematology		Reference Range
PCV (%)	29	24–45
NCC (×10³/µl)	2	5.5–19.5
NRBC (×10³/µl)	0.1	0
Segs (×10³/µl)	11.6	2.5–12.5
Bands (×10³/µl)	0.1	0–0.3
Monos (×10³/µl)	0.4	0–0.8
Lymphs (×10³/µl)	0.7	1.5–7
Eos (×10³/µl)	0.8	0–1.5
Platelets (×10³/µl)	304	150–700

Morphology: Many acanthocyte-like RBCs, occasional fragmented RBC

Biochemical Profile		Reference Range
Gluc (mg/dl)	67	67–124 (3.7–6.8 mmol/L)
BUN (mg/dl)	14	17–32 (6.1–11.4 mmol/L)
Creat (mg/dl)	1.2	0.9–2.1
Ca (mg/dl)	9.0	8.5–11
Phos (mg/dl)	5.1	3.3–7.8
TP (g/dl)	6.2	5.9–8.1
Alb (g/dl)	3.0	2.3–3.9
T. Bili (mg/dl)	6.3 (108)	0–0.3 (0–5.1 µmol/L)
ALT (IU/L)	332	30–100
ALP (IU/L)	2185	11–210
Na (mEq/L)	149	146–160
K (mEq/L)	5.2	3.7–5.4
CL (mEq/L)	109	112–129
TCO₂ (mEq/L)	19	14–23

Interpretive Discussion

Hematology

The hematocrit is low normal. The leukogram shows a lymphopenia with a high normal concentration of mature neutrophils; this is interpreted as a stress or steroid leukogram. There are acanthocyte-like or spiculated cells present. These are commonly observed in cats with liver disease or hepatic lipidosis.

Biochemical Profile

The mildly decreased BUN may be insignificant or may be due to decreased hepatic urea production or decreased protein intake. The combination of hyperbilirubinemia and increased ALT and ALP activities is characteristic of hepatic lipidosis in cats. The combination of hepatocellular injury (indicated by increased ALT) and cholestasis (indicated by increased ALP) lead to failure of bilirubin clearance and hyperbilirubinemia. This degree of increase in ALP activity is unusual in cats, other than in association with hepatic lipidosis. Lipidosis is thought to occur as a result of massive fat mobilization from adipocytes in association with anorexia of several days duration or acute diabetes.

Summary

The biochemical findings are characteristic of hepatic lipidosis, which was conformed by liver aspiration cytology.

CASE 43

Signalment: 7-year-old female Border collie
History: Depression, anorexia
Physical Examination: Ascites, dermatitis of face and genital area

Hematology		Reference Range
PCV (%)	15	37–55
MCV (fl)	57	60–72
Retics (/µl)	118	<60
NCC (×10³/µl)	9.5	6–17
Segs (×10³/µl)	4.3	3–11.5
Bands (×10³/µl)	2.2	0–0.3
Metas (×10³/µl)	0.6	0
Monos (×10³/µl)	0.8	0.1–1.3
Lymphs (×10³/µl)	0.7	1–4.8
NRBC (×10³/µl)	0.9	0
Platelets (×10³/µl)	20	200–500

Hemopathology: target cells, acanthocytes, schistocytes, toxic neutrophils, giant platelets

Biochemical Profile		Reference Range
Gluc (mg/dl)	45	65–122
BUN (mg/dl)	16	7–28
Creat (mg/dl)	1.0	0.9–1.7
Ca (mg/dl)	9.2	9.0–11.2
Phos (mg/dl)	3.8	2.8–6.1
TP (g/dl)	4.5	5.4–7.4
Alb (g/dl)	1.7	2.7–4.5
Glob (g/dl)	2.8	1.9–3.4
T. Bili (mg/dl)	3.3	0–0.4
Chol (mg/dl)	86	130–370
ALP (IU)	1391	35–280
ALT (IU)	239	10–120
Na (mEq/L)	147	145–158
K (mEq/L)	2.6	4.1–5.5
CL (mEq/L)	122	106–127
TCO₂ (mEq/L)	8.5	14–27

Fluid Analysis (abdominal)	
Color	Straw
Transparency	Clear
NCC (/µl)	1300
TP (g/dl)	1.5

Coagulation Data		
PT (sec)	20	6.5–9.0
aPTT (sec)	36	12–16

Interpretive Discussion

Hematology

PCV is decreased, indicating anemia. Reticulocytes are increased, indicating that the anemia is somewhat regenerative. MCV is decreased, particularly in light of increased reticulocytes, suggesting iron deficiency anemia secondary to chronic blood loss.

Inflammatory leukogram is present, as evidenced by the marked left shift. In light of low number of segmented neutrophils, sepsis or endotoxemia may be present. Lymphopenia suggests a stress leukogram.

Thrombocytopenia and the presence of schistocytes as well as prolonged PT and APTT suggest disseminated intravascular coagulopathy (DIC).

Biochemical Profile

Hypoglycemia may be due to sepsis (leukogram is suggestive of sepsis or endotoxemia), end-stage liver disease, insulinoma, or other type of neoplasia, such as a large hepatoma.

Hypoalbuminemia, in conjunction with low cholesterol, is indicative of GI disease (malabsorption, maldigestion, protein losing enteropathy) or end-stage liver disease. Another possible cause of low total protein is blood loss, since MCV indicates iron deficiency anemia. However, albumin is relatively lower than globulin.

Total bilirubin is increased. While the animal is anemic, and blood destruction is a possible cause, the MCV suggests blood loss. Therefore the bilirubin is probably increased due to cholestasis or hepatocellular dysfunction. Increased alkaline phosphatase activity suggests cholestasis.

Cholesterol is decreased, likely due to end-stage liver disease (see hypoalbuminemia discussion).

Hypokalemia may be due to decreased intake. In face of acidosis, it indicates total body depletion.

Decreased total CO_2 indicates metabolic acidosis. The decrease is likely due to lactic acidosis in this patient, since the dog is not uremic and there is no evidence of diabetic ketoacidosis.

Abdominal Fluid Analysis

Transudate, likely due to liver disease and hypoalbuminemia.

Coagulation Data

While prolonged PT and APPT may be due to lack of synthesis of coagulation factors by the liver, another explanation is DIC, in light of the decreased platelets.

Summary

End-stage liver disease; cholestasis
DIC
Inflammation, possibly sepsis
Iron deficiency anemia

Dermatitis was determined to be necrolytic migratory erythema (superficial necrolytic dermatitis), which is associated with hyperglucagonemia, often seen with severe hepatic disease (hepatocutaneous syndrome).

CASE 44

Signalment: 10-year-old spayed female miniature schnauzer

History: Polydipsia, polyuria, weight loss, abdominal "cramping" for 1 month

Physical Examination: Tense abdomen, thin with mild truncal alopecia and comedones on dorsal midline

Hematology		Reference Range
PCV (%)	48	37–55
NCC (×10³/µl)	**34.4**	6–17
Segs (×10³/µl)	**29.0**	3–11.5
Bands (×10³/µl)	**2.0**	0–0.3
Monos (×10³/µl)	**3.4**	0.1–1.3
Lymphs (×10³/µl)	0	1–4.8
Platelets (×10³/µl)	Adequate	200–500
TP (P) (g/dl)	**9.0***	6–8

*although dog fasted, plasma is markedly lipemic, so refractometric measurement of total protein may be falsely increased

Biochemical Profile		Reference Range
Gluc (mg/dl)	**353 (19.4)**	65–122 (3.7–6.8 mmol/L)
BUN (mg/dl)	**35 (12.5)**	7–28 (6.1–11.4 mmol/L)
Creat (mg/dl)	1.2	0.9–1.7
Ca (mg/dl)	11.0	9.0–11.2
Phos (mg/dl)	6.0	2.8–6.1
TP (g/dl)	6.0	5.4–7.4
Alb (g/dl)	2.7	2.7–4.5
Glob (g/dl)	3.3	1.9–3.4
T. Bili (mg/dl)	**1.2 (26.5)**	0–0.4 (0–6.8 µmol/L)
Chol (mg/dl)	**900 (23.4)**	130–370 (3.4–9.6 mmol/L)
ALT (IU/L)	**987**	10–120
ALP (IU/L)	**1200**	35–280
Na (mEq/L)	**139**	145–158
K (mEq/L)	**3.1**	4.1–5.5
CL (mEq/L)	**100**	106–127
TCO₂ (mEq/L)	**12.2**	14–27
An. gap (mEq/L)	**30**	8–25
Lipase (IU/L)	**3500**	30–560

Urinalysis	
Color	Yellow
Transparency	Clear
Sp. Gr.	1.035
Protein	Neg
Gluc	2+
Ketones	Neg
Bilirubin	+
Blood	Neg
pH	6.0

Endocrine Data		Reference Range
ACTH stimulation:		
serum cortisol (µg/dl)(pre)	**4.5 (124)**	1–4 (28–110 nmol/L)
serum cortisol (µg/dl)(post)	14.6	<20
Low dose dexamethasone suppression test:		
serum cortisol (µg/dl)(pre)	3.5	1–4
serum cortisol (µg/dl)(8-hour post)	1.5	<1.5

Interpretive Discussion

Hematology

Lymphopenia is indicative of increased endogenous (stress or hyperadrenocorticism) or exogenous corticosteroids. Increased immature neutrophil concentration is indicative of inflammation. Neutrophilia may be due to inflammation or stress. In summary, an inflammatory and stress (steroid) leukogram is present.

Biochemical Profile

Hyperglycemia is of the magnitude that diabetes mellitus should be suspected. Hyperglycemia may also be secondary to hyperadrenocorticism; therefore, adrenocorticotropic hormone (ACTH) stimulation and low dose dexamethasone suppression tests (LDDS) are indicated.

BUN is increased, but creatinine is within the reference range. Urine specific gravity indicates kidneys are capable of concentrating, thus the azotemia is prerenal, perhaps due to dehydration. However, albumin is within reference range. The PCV is normal, suggesting that GI bleeding is not the cause of the increased BUN.

Total bilirubin is increased suggesting cholestasis, because anemia is not present. Alkaline phosphatase activity is increased, which is also suggestive of cholestasis. Another consideration is hyperadrenocorticism, with an increase in the corticosteroid-induced alkaline phosphatase isoenzyme. Increased cholesterol of this magnitude is most likely due to lipemia, although some component of the increase could also be due to cholestasis. ALT activity is increased, which is indicative of hepatocellular damage.

Sodium and chloride concentrations are decreased. Sodium may be lost through the kidney, although this animal is capable of concentrating. Although it is not mentioned in the history, abdominal pain may have been associated with vomiting, which would result in electrolyte loss. Hyperglycemia results in increased serum osmolality with a shift of intracellular fluid to extracellular fluid in an attempt to decrease extracellular fluid solute concentration. Sodium can be expected to decrease by 1.6 mEq/L for every 100 mg/dl increase in glucose.

Total CO_2 is decreased, indicating metabolic acidosis. The anion gap is increased, indicating increased unmeasured anions are present. In this case, unmeasured anions might be ketones, although they are not present in the urine. Other possibilities include lactic acidosis.

Serum lipase activity is increased. In this patient, this increase could partially be due to decreased GFR, as indicated by azotemia. However, inflammatory leukogram, increased bilirubin, increased alkaline phosphatase activity, hyperglycemia, and lipemia are also suggestive of pancreatitis. This magnitude of lipase increase is highly supportive of pancreatitis. Prerenal azotemia due to hemoconcentration and poor renal perfusion is a common complication of pancreatitis. Likewise, so is hepatocellular injury and cholestasis.

Urinalysis

Urine specific gravity of 1.035 indicates the dog is capable of concentrating, thus the increase in BUN is prerenal (perhaps dehydration). Glucosuria and bilirubinuria are to be expected in light of the serum concentrations.

Endocrine Data

ACTH stimulation test: Baseline cortisol is slightly above normal. Normal animals stimulate to around 10 to 16 μg/dl. Low dose dexamethasone suppression test: Baseline cortisol is normal. Dog suppressed marginally at 8 hours. The endocrine data are not supportive of hyperadrenocorticism.

Summary

This dog has primary hyperlipidemia, which has been shown to be familial in miniature schnauzers (Rogers WA, EF Donovan, GJ Kociba. Idiopathic hyperlipoproteinemia in dogs. J Am Vet Med Assoc 1975;166:1087–1091), and pancreatitis with secondary diabetes mellitus. Dogs with hyperlipidemia are predisposed to development of pancreatitis. While diabetes mellitus may be transitory, treatment is indicated. Some abnormalities (hyperglycemia, stress leukogram, increased alkaline phosphatase activity, lipemia, history, and physical appearance) were suggestive of hyperadrenocorticism. This possibility was ruled out by the ACTH stimulation and LDDS test. Imaging revealed evidence of swelling in the area of the pancreas.

CASE 45

Signalment: 9-year-old SF canine, miniature schnauzer
History: Not eating, vomited a few times
Physical Examination: Tense abdomen

Hematology		Reference Range
PCV (%)	**32.0**	37–55
MCV (fl)	68.0	60–72
NCC (×10³/µl)	**5.2**	6–17
Segs (×10³/µl)	**2.7**	3–11.5
Bands (×10³/µl)	**1.4**	0–0.3
Monos (×10³/µl)	0.2	0.1–1.3
Lymphs (×10³/µl)	**0.6**	1–4.8
Basophils (×10³/µl)	0.1	rare
Platelets (×10³/µl)	**111**	200–500

Hemopathology: marked toxic neutrophils, giant platelets, hemolyzed and lipemic

Biochemical Profile		Reference Range
Gluc (mg/dl)	**226 (12.4)**	65–122 *(3.5–6.7 mmol/L)*
BUN (mg/dl)	20	7–28
Creat (mg/dl)	1.2	0.9–1.7
Ca (mg/dl)	**8.2 (2.0)**	9.0–11.2 *(2.2–2.8 mmol/L)*
Phos (mg/dl)	5.1	2.8–6.1
TP (g/dl)	**5.0**	5.4–7.4
Alb (g/dl)	**1.8**	2.7–4.5
Glob (g/dl)	3.2	1.9–3.4
T. Bili (mg/dl)	**1.4 (23.9)**	0–0.4 *(0.6–8.4 µmol/L)*
Chol (mg/dl)	**666 (17.3)**	130–370 *(3.4–9.6 mmol/L)*
ALT (IU/L)	33	10–120
AST (IU/L)	51	16–40
ALP (IU/L)	**1282**	35–280
GGT (IU/L)	5	0–6
Na (mEq/L)	152	145–158
K (mEq/L)	**3.7**	4.1–5.5
CL (mEq/L)	116	106–127
TCO₂ (mEq/L)	14	14–27
An. gap (mEq/L)	25	8–25
Amylase (IU/L)	**2421**	50–1250
Lipase (IU/L)	**2256**	30–560
Triglycerides (mg/dl)	**2884**	ND*

* Not Determined

Urinalysis			
Color	Golden	**Urine Sediment**	
Transparency	Cloudy	WBCs/hpf	2–3
Sp. Gr.	1.034	RBCs/hpf	3–5
Protein	**2+**	Epith cells/hpf	Negative
Gluc	**4+**	Casts/lpf	2
Bilirubin	**3+**	Crystals	Negative
Blood	**2+**	Bacteria	Negative
pH	8.0		
ketones	Negative		

Coagulation Data		Reference Range
PT (seconds)	9.3	7.5–10.5
aPTT (seconds)	**19.5**	10.5–16.5

Abdominal Fluid Analysis	
Color	Red
Supernatant	Light yellow
Refractometric protein (g/dl)	**7.2**
NCC (×10³/µl)	2.0
Triglyceride (mg/dl)	**257**
Chol (mg/dl)	**728**

Interpretive Discussion

HematologyThe PCV is mildly decreased, no polychromasia was noted in the blood film, and the MCV is normal, indicating a mild nonregenerative anemia. Marked lipemia and hemolysis may have resulted in *in vitro* hemolysis, but this typically does not result in an important decrease in the PCV. There is a neutropenia with increased bands and marked numbers of toxic neutrophils. This suggests consumption as a result of severe inflammatory disease. Lymphopenia indicates a stress component. The thrombocytopenia is discussed with the coagulation data.

Biochemical Profile

The serum glucose concentration is moderately increased. In this range, it is possible that this is a stress hyperglycemia, but is more likely due to some metabolic or endocrine abnormality.

The BUN and serum creatinine concentrations are normal. The serum phosphorus is normal, but there is a mild decrease in serum total calcium concentration. Given the degree of hypoalbuminemia, it is wise to attempt to correct the total calcium for the hypoproteinemia. In this case, the corrected value is 9.9 mg/dl (8.2–1.8 + 3.5), which is normal.

The serum cholesterol concentration is markedly increased. While this may be associated with cholestasis, given the degree of increase in cholesterol one should also consider other metabolic abnormalities including hepatic disease, disorders of lipoprotein metabolism, or endocrinopathies. The serum triglyceride concentration is markedly increased, and further supports a diagnosis of a metabolic and/or endocrinologic disorder. Cholestasis is indicated by the increased total bilirubin and ALP activity. The serum ALT, AST, and GGT activities are normal or near normal, reducing the likelyhood of hepatocellular injury.

The serum amylase and lipase activities are significantly increased, and in the absence of azotemia suggest acute pancreatitis. This is a frequent complication of severe prolonged hyperlipidemia. The concurrent findings of hyperlipidemia and pancreatitis in a miniature schnauzer should alert one to the potential diagnosis of a primary dyslipidemia.

Coagulation Data

The coagulation profile includes a normal PT, but prolonged APTT. While it is more common for the PT to become prolonged first when there is impaired coagulation factor synthesis by the liver, incipient DIC (note the thrombocytopenia) or heparinization of the patient may result in changes in the APTT alone.

Abdominal Fluid Analysis

Abdominal fluid chemical analysis similarly indicates accumulation of excess lipids in the peritoneal cavity. It is likely that the increased total protein by refractometry is spuriously elevated by this lipid. The cell concentration suggests a modified transudate.

Urinalysis

The urinary specific gravity is normal, and the number of leukocytes and erythrocytes are not significant. However, there is 2+ proteinuria, some occult blood, and some hyaline and fine granular casts. Thus, there may be tubular disease. In addition, there is significant glucosuria, which is explained by the hyperglycemia. It would be useful to evaluate the UPC in order to determine the magnitude of the proteinuria. Given the hypoalbuminemia and hypercholesterolemia, one should consider the possibility of nephrotic syndrome; there may be a protein-losing glomerulopathy without azotemia.

Summary

Minature schnauzer hyperlipidemia and acute pancreatitis.

CASE 46

Signalment: 11-year-old castrated male cat

History: Polyuria and polydipsia for 2 months. Anorexia and lethargy more recently.

Physical Examination: Presented in lateral recumbency. 10% dehydrated.

Hematology		Reference Range
PCV (%)	40	24–45
Hgb (g/dl)	12.8	8–15
RBC (×10⁶/µl)	8.64	5–11
MCV (fl)	46	39–50
MCHC (g/dl)	34	33–37
NCC (×10³/µl)	18.7	5.5–19.5
Segs (×10³/µl)	**15.0**	2.5–12.5
Bands (×10³/µl)	**2.4**	0–0.3
Monos (×10³/µl)	0.2	0–0.8
Lymphs (×10³/µl)	**0.9**	1.5–7.0
Eos (×10³/µl)	0.2	0–1.5
Platelets (×10³/µl)	375	150–700
TP (P) (g/dl)	**11.7**	6–8

Hemopathology: Slightly toxic neutrophils, many echinocytes.

Biochemical Profile		Reference Range
Gluc (mg/dl)	**766 (42.7)**	67–124 (3.7–6.8 mmol/L)
BUN (mg/dl)	**127 (45.3)**	17–32 (6.1–11.4 mmol/L)
Creat (mg/dl)	**6.4 (566)**	0.9–2.1 (78–186 µmol/L)
Ca (mg/dl)	10.1	8.5–11
Phos (mg/dl)	**7.9 (10.0)**	3.3–7.8 (1.1–2.5 mmol/L)
TP (g/dl)	**9.7**	5.9–8.1
Alb (g/dl)	**4.4**	2.3–3.9
Glob (g/dl)	**5.3**	2.9–4.4
T. Bili (mg/dl)	0.3	0–0.3
Chol (mg/dl)	**388 (10.1)**	60–220 (1.6–5.7 mmol/L)
ALT (IU/L)	**124**	30–100
AST (IU/L)	**354**	14–38
ALP (IU/L)	65	6–106
GGT (IU/L)	1	0–1
Na (mEq/L)	**172**	146–160
K (mEq/L)	5.1	3.7–5.4
CL (mEq/L)	**132**	112–129
TCO₂ (mEq/L)	**10.9**	14–23
An. gap (mEq/L)	**34**	10–27
Calc. Osmolarity (mOsm/L)	**417**	290–310

Urinalysis (cystocentesis)			
Color	Yellow	**Urine Sediment**	
Transparency	Cloudy	WBCs/hpf	**6–8**
Sp. Gr.	1.034	RBCs/hpf	2–3
Protein	**2+**	Epith cells/hpf	1–3 transitional
Gluc	**2+**	Casts/lpf	0
Bilirubin	Negative	Crystals	0
Blood	**4+**	Bacteria	0
pH	5.0	Ketones	Negative
		Other	Small amt of fat

Interpretive Discussion

Hematology

Leukogram abnormalities include neutrophilia, a left shift, lymphopenia, and slightly toxic neutrophils. This is an inflammatory leukogram indicating a tissue demand for neutrophils. The lymphopenia suggests concurrent increase in corticosteroid concentrations due to stress. Toxic neutrophils indicate a rapid rate of neutrophil production.

Echinocyte formation can be an artefact, but in this case, it may have resulted from the marked hyperosmolality and electrolyte abnormalities. These may have caused movement of water from the cytoplasm of erythrocytes to the plasma with resulting shrinkage and crenation of erythrocytes.

Biochemical Profile

The serum glucose concentration is markedly increased. The most likely cause of hyperglycemia of this magnitude is diabetes mellitus. Severe, acute excitement with release of catecholamines can cause marked hyperglycemia in cats, but serum glucose concentration is seldom greater than 400 mg/dl in such cats. This cat is azotemic, and decreased renal excretion of glucose, secondary to decreased glomerular filtration rate, may have augmented the magnitude of the hyperglycemia.

Both BUN and serum creatinine concentrations are increased. Since the urine specific gravity suggests adequate renal concentrating ability (i.e., the specific gravity is greater than 1.030), this appears to be a prerenal azotemia. However, the marked hyperproteinemia and hypernatremia suggest severe dehydration, and an even higher urine specific gravity would be expected in this situation. It is, therefore, possible that this cat has some loss of urine concentration ability. Alternatively, osmotic diuresis due to glucosuria may have contributed to the lower than expected urine specific gravity. The hyperphosphatemia is a result of a decreased glomerular filtration rate. Maintenance of normal serum phosphorus concentrations depends on phosphorus excretion through glomeruli.

Hyperproteinemia (both plasma and serum protein) with concurrent hyperalbuminemia and hyperglobulinemia is typical of dehydration. Contraction of plasma water volume results in proportional increases in concentrations of both albumin and globulin. Although other abnormalities can cause hyperglobulinemia, dehydration is the only cause of hyperalbuminemia. Diuresis secondary to glucosuria is common in diabetes mellitus and can result in dehydration.

The serum cholesterol concentration is increased. In this case, this abnormality is probably secondary to diabetes mellitus and related abnormalities in lipid metabolism.

Serum activities of both ALT and AST are increased. The increased serum ALT activity is due to hepatocyte injury and subsequent leakage of this enzyme. This injury was probably caused by fatty change which developed secondary to the metabolic abnormalities of diabetes mellitus. The increased serum AST activity may also be due to leakage of AST from injured hepatocytes, but the higher activity of AST as compared to ALT suggests that there is also an extrahepatic source. This source may be muscle, and may have resulted from muscle injury secondary to hypoperfusion, since the cat is very dehydrated.

Hypernatremia and hyperchloremia are probably due to severe dehydration. Glucosuria causes diuresis resulting in Na and Cl loss through the kidneys in nondehydrated or mildly dehydrated, diabetic animals. This can lead to hyponatremia and hypochloremia. When such animals become severely dehydrated, however, diuresis no longer occurs, and hypernatremia and hyperchloremia develop. These changes, in combination with hyperglycemia and azotemia, result in severe hyperosmolality.

Decreased serum total CO_2 concentration probably represents a primary metabolic acidosis. Serum total CO_2 concentration may also decrease as a compensatory reaction in animals with primary respiratory alkalosis, but in animals with diabetes mellitus, metabolic acidosis is more likely to be the primary alteration. Increased serum concentrations of ketones are a common cause of acidosis in diabetic animals, but the absence of urine ketones suggests that this cat is probably not ketotic. Urine ketone tests that use the nitroprusside reaction do not detect β-hydroxybutyric acid, therefore, the presence of this ketone cannot be ruled out. Increased serum lactate concentration may be contributing to the acidosis in this cat. The cat is markedly dehydrated and is, therefore, probably experiencing tissue hypoxia which may lead to increased lactate production.

The anion gap is increased. In most diabetic animals, increased ketoacid concentration in the blood is the major cause of this abnormality. In this cat, which is apparently not ketotic, increased blood lactate concentration is probably contributing to this gap.

The calculated osmolarity is increased and, in combination with other laboratory changes, suggests this cat has diabetic nonketotic hyperosmolar syndrome (see summary).

Urinalysis

This cat has a proteinuria with a mild pyuria. It is possible that the protein exuded into the urine as part of the inflammatory process; however, the degree of proteinuria appears to be excessive compared to the degree of pyuria. Other causes of proteinuria such as glomerular and tubular disease should be considered in this case. Although glomerular disease has been associated with diabetes mellitus in humans, this has not been documented in animals.

The strongly positive reaction on the chemical test for blood in combination with normal numbers of erythrocytes suggests that the positive reaction is due to either free hemoglobin or myoglobin. It is unlikely that this represents a hematuria with subsequent lysis of erythrocytes since such lysis is unlikely in urine with a high specific gravity. Absence of anemia suggests a significant hemolytic problem is not occurring in this cat. Myoglobinuria is a possible explanation, and severe muscle hypoxia secondary to hypovolemia may have occurred in this cat. However, the serum AST activity, while increased, does not suggest such massive muscle injury.

Glucosuria is a result of the serum glucose concentration exceeding the renal threshold.

Summary

The clinical diagnosis was diabetic nonketotic hyperosmolar syndrome. This syndrome is characterized by marked hyperglycemia (blood glucose concentration > 600 mg/dl), hyperosmolarity (>350 mOsm/l), and absence of ketosis in a diabetic animal. Such animals commonly have prerenal or renal azotemia. The hyperosmolarity results in dehydration of neurons and subsequent neurologic signs. This syndrome is associated with a high fatality rate.

After a brief, unsuccessful attempt to decrease serum glucose concentrations with insulin therapy and to improve the cat's electrolyte and fluid balance by administration of fluids, the owner elected euthanasia. Necropsy revealed severe islet cell degeneration and amyloidosis and severe hepatocytic vacuolar degeneration. A few mineralized casts were present in renal tubules, but the kidneys were otherwise normal, and the azotemia was probably prerenal in this case. The cause of the inflammatory leukogram was not determined.

CASE 47

Signalment: 10-year-old MC feline DSH
History: Not eating well, lethargic
Physical Examination: Slightly dehydrated

Hematology	Day 1	Reference Range
PCV (%)	38.0*	24–45
Hgb (g/dl)	12.8	8–15
RBC (×10⁶/µl)	9.25	5–11
MCV (fl)	44.0	39–50
MCHC (g/dl)	35.0	33–37
NCC (×10³/µl)	12.9	5.5–19.5
Segs (×10³/µl)	12.5	2.5–12.5
Lymphs (×10³/µl)	**0.3**	1.5–7.0
Platelets (×10³/µl)	Adequate	150–700
TP (P) (g/dl)	**9.0**	6–8

Hemopathology: giant platelets, slight increase in polychromasia, slt toxic neutrophils, **2+ Heinz bodies**

* PCV was 27% on Day 5, and 17% on Day 7.

Biochemical Profile	Day 1	Reference Range
Gluc (mg/dl)	**328 (18.0)**	67–124 (3.7–6.8 mmol/L)
BUN (mg/dl)	29	17–32
Creat (mg/dl)	1.5	0.9–2.1
Ca (mg/dl)	9.4	8.5–11
Phos (mg/dl)	**1.9 (0.6)**	3.3–7.8 (1.1–2.5 mmol/L)
TP (g/dl)	8.0	5.9–8.1
Alb (g/dl)	**4.3**	2.3–3.9
Glob (g/dl)	3.7	2.9–4.4
T. Bili (mg/dl)	**2.1 (35.9)**	0–0.3 (0–5.1 µmol/L)
Chol (mg/dl)	**512 (13.3)**	60–220 (1.6–5.7 mmol/L)
ALT (IU/L)	**282**	30–100
ALP (IU/L)	99	6–106
Na (mEq/L)	**130**	146–160
K (mEq/L)	**2.2**	3.7–5.4
CL (mEq/L)	**74**	112–129
TCO₂ (mEq/L)	**10.5**	14–23
An. gap (mEq/L)	**47.7**	10–27
Lipase (IU/L)	**161**	3–125

Blood Gas Data (arterial)		Reference Range
pH	**7.280**	7.33–7.44
PCO₂ (mmHg)	**20.0**	35–42
PO₂ (mmHg)	85.5	73–92
HCO₃ (mEq/L)	**9.2**	16–22
ionized Ca++ (mg/dl)	**4.64**	4.8–5.3

Urinalysis

Color	Yellow	Urine Sediment	
Transparency	Clear	WBCs/hpf	0–1
Sp. Gr.	1.033	RBCs/hpf	0–1
Protein	1+	Epith cells/hpf	0–1
Gluc	4+	Casts/lpf	**3–4 granular**
Bilirubin	1+	Crystals	Negative
Blood	1+	Bacteria	Negative
pH	6.0	Other	
Ketones	**3+**		

Interpretive Discussion

Hematology

The packed cell volume, hemoglobin, and total RBC count are normal, but given the degree of hemoconcentration represented by the hyperproteinemia, it is possible that the PCV is actually lower. There is a slight increase in polychromasia. The anemia is rapidly progressive over a 1 week period of time. The presence of 2+ Heinz bodies indicates significant oxidative damage to the red blood cells, and is commonly observed in cats with diabetes mellitus. Another potential cause of hemolytic anemia in this patient is hypophosphatemia. There is a stress leukogram, as indicated by the high normal neutrophil count and lymphopenia.

Biochemical Profile

The serum glucose concentration is moderately increased. While a glucose concentration of this magnitude may be encountered due to extreme excitement (sympathetic activation) or stress (glucocorticoid release), diabetes mellitus is more likely. The BUN and serum creatinine concentrations are normal.

The serum phosphorus concentration is decreased, and given the degree of hyperglycemia, one should consider diabetic ketoacidosis-induced urinary phosphate loss. The serum total calcium concentration is normal, reducing the possibility of an endocrine abnormality causing the change in serum phosphorus. The serum total protein concentration is at the upper end of the reference range, and serum albumin is increased, indicating hemoconcentration due to dehydration.

The serum cholesterol concentration is moderately increased. While this may be associated with cholestasis, as indicated by the increased total bilirubin, the ALP activity is normal. Given the degree of increase in cholesterol, one should consider metabolic abnormalities including hepatic disease, disorders of lipoprotein metabolism, or endocrinopathies. If not due to cholestasis, then the increase in bilirubin may be due to hemolysis. The serum ALT activity is increased modestly which indicates hepatocellular damage. ALP is not induced by steroids in cats, thus, hyperadrenocorticism is a possibility. Serum lipase activity is only slightly increased, possibly reducing the probability for concurrent pancreatitis; however, increased lipase activity is not a good marker for feline pancreatitis.

Serum Na, K, and Cl concentration are decreased significantly. One should consider typical causes for electrolyte depletion, including pathologic losses from the gastrointestinal and urinary systems, as well as a shift to third space. The marked hyperglycemia should initiate consideration of diabetic ketoacidosis with subsequent urinary electrolyte loss. There is a marked decrease in serum total CO_2 suggesting metabolic acidosis. The increase in the anion gap is likely due to the presence of ketones, which act as unmeasured anions.

Blood Gas Data

The blood gas panel indicates a metabolic acidosis (decreased pH and HCO_3) with respiratory compensation (decreased pCO_2). Ionized calcium is marginally decreased.

Urinalysis

The urinary specific gravity is normal. However, with marked increases in the concentration of solutes, such as glucose, not pertinent to urinary concentration capacity, one might question the accuracy of this measure, and consider determining urinary osmolality to address urinary concentration capacity specifically. The presence of 1+ protein and coarse granular casts is consistent with renal tubular disease. The absence of more significant proteinuria speaks against the possibility of glomerular protein loss, but a urinary protein:creatinine ratio should be determined to confirm this. In either case, urinary tract inflammation is not a likely cause of the observed changes, as there is only a small amount of occult blood and no pyuria. The presence of significant amounts of glucose and ketones supports a diagnosis of diabetic ketoacidosis. The mild bilirubinuria is a result of the increased serum bilirubin and subsequent renal excretion.

Summary

Diabetic ketoacidosis; Heinz body anemia

CASE 48

Signalment: 3-year-old castrated male golden retriever
History: Lethargic, heat seeking
Physical Examination: Obese, poor hair coat, tailhead alopecia

Hematology		Reference Range
PCV (%)	**34**	37–55
MCV (fl)	65	60–72
MCHC (g/dl)	35	34–38
Retics (/µl)	**2**	<60
NCC (×10³/µl)	12.5	6–17
Segs (×10³/µl)	9.3	3–11.5
Monos (×10³/µl)	1.0	0.1–1.3
Lymphs (×10³/µl)	2.2	1–4.8
Platelets (×10³/µl)	Adequate	200–500
TP (P) (g/dl)	7.5	6–8

Hemopathology: Numerous leptocytes ("target cells") present

Biochemical Profile		Reference Range
Gluc (mg/dl)	105	65–122
BUN (mg/dl)	20	7–28
Creat (mg/dl)	1.2	0.9–1.7
Ca (mg/dl)	10.5	9.0–11.2
Phos (mg/dl)	4.0	2.8–6.1
TP (g/dl)	7.0	5.4–7.4
Alb (g/dl)	3.7	2.7–4.5
Glob (g/dl)	3.3	1.9–3.4
T. Bili (mg/dl)	0.2	0–0.4
Chol (mg/dl)	**720 (18.7)**	130–370 (3.4–9.6 mmol/L)
ALT (IU/L)	110	10–120
AST (IU/L)	35	16–40
ALP (IU/L)	220	35–280
Na (mEq/L)	**143**	145–158
K (mEq/L)	4.5	4.1–5.5
CL (mEq/L)	107	106–127
TCO₂ (mEq/L)	20	14–27

Endocrine Data		Reference Range
TT4 (µg/dl)	1.6	1.4–4.0
Free T4 (ng/dl)	**0.24 (3.0)**	1.2–3.4 (15.4–43.8 pmol/L)
Endogenous TSH (ng/ml) (Immulite)	**0.5**	0.1–0.45

Interpretive Discussion

Hematology

A mild nonregenerative, normocytic, normochromic anemia is the only abnormality in the CBC. "Target cells" are common and are not very diagnostically useful. They are commonly present in animals with hypercholesterolemia.

Biochemical Profile

The only abnormalities present are hypercholesterolemia and mild hyponatremia. Hypercholesterolemia is marked, and in conjunction with the history, physical examination, and mild anemia, is very suggestive of hypothyroidism. Mild hyponatremia has been reported in approximately 30% of dogs with hypothyroidism.

Endocrine Data

Total T4 is within the reference range. However, since many variables affect TT4, and this dog has clinical and laboratory findings that are suggestive of hypothyroidism, a free T4 and endogenous TSH are indicated. The decreased FT4 and increased endogenous TSH are diagnostic for hypothyroidism.

Summary

Early primary hypothyroidism.

CASE 49

Signalment: 3-year-old MC English springer spaniel
History: Anorexia, occasional vomiting
Physical Examination: Lethargic, thin, approximately 8% dehydrated

Hematology		Reference Range
PCV (%)	**32**	37–55
Hgb (g/dl)	**11.1**	12–18
RBC (×10⁶/µl)	**4.47**	5.5–8.5
MCV (fl)	72	60–72
MCHC (g/dl)	35	34–38
Retics (/µl)	ND*	<60
NCC (×10³/µl)	9.8	6–17
Segs (×10³/µl)	5.6	3–11.5
Monos (×10³/µl)	0.8	0.1–1.3
Lymphs (×10³/µl)	2.2	1.0–4.8
Eos (×10³/µl)	1.2	0.1–1.2
Platelets (×10³/µl)	Adequate	200–500
TP (P) (g/dl)	**8.5**	6–8

* Not Determined

Biochemical Profile		Reference Range
Gluc (mg/dl)	83	65–122
BUN (mg/dl)	**47 (16.8)**	7–28 (2.5–10.0 mmol/L)
Creat (mg/dl)	1.6	0.9–1.7
Ca (mg/dl)	**13.8 (3.45)**	9.0–11.2 (2.25–2.80 mmol/L)
Phos (mg/dl)	**6.2 (2.0)**	2.8–6.1 (0.9–2.0 mmol/L)
TP (g/dl)	**7.5**	5.4–7.4
Alb (g/dl)	**5.0**	2.7–4.5
Glob (g/dl)	2.5	1.9–3.4
T. Bili (mg/dl)	0.2	0–0.4
Chol (mg/dl)	135	130–370
ALT (IU/L)	49	10–120
AST (IU/L)	19	16–40
ALP (IU/L)	98	35–280
Na (mEq/L)	**132**	145–158
K (mEq/L)	5.5	4.1–5.5
CL (mEq/L)	**97**	106–127
TCO₂ (mEq/L)	**10**	14–27
An. gap (mEq/L)	**30**	8–25
Amylase (IU/L)	1300	50–1250
Lipase (IU/L)	570	30–560

Endocrine Data		Reference Range
ACTH stimulation		
serum cortisol (µg/dl)(pre)	**<0.1 (<2.8)**	1–4 (28–110 nmol/L)
serum cortisol (µg/dl)(post)	**<0.1 (<2.8)**	<10.5 (<290 nmol/L)

Urinalysis	
Urine specific gravity	1.020

Interpretive Discussion

Hematology

A mild anemia is present. Reticulocyte concentration was not determined, thus the degree of regeneration is unknown. Increased polychromasia is not mentioned, suggesting that the anemia is nonregenerative; however, the MCV is at the upper end of the reference range, suggesting the presence of large immature erythrocytes. Considering the degree of dehydration, anemia is likely more severe than is apparent.

While the leukogram is normal, a patient that is ill and vomiting would be expected to have a stress leukogram. The absence of a stress leukogram should prompt consideration of hypoadrenocorticism.

Plasma protein is increased, probably as a result of dehydration.

Biochemical Profile

Azotemia is evidenced by increased BUN, creatinine, and phosphorus concentrations. While azotemia may be pre-renal, since the dog is dehydrated, one would expect the urine specific gravity to be greater than 1.030, if this were the case. However, the serum sodium concentration is decreased, and ability to concentrate is impaired by medullary washout of sodium. Refer to the discussion on sodium and potassium for further interpretation.

Hypercalcemia, in light of hyponatremia and hyperkalemia, is likely due to hypoadrenocorticism. The pathophysiology may be related to decreased glucocorticoids and subsequent increased GI calcium uptake, calcium retention by the kidney, as related to sodium loss, or increased albumin-bound calcium. Other causes of hypercalcemia, such as hypercalcemia of malignancy, primary hyperparathyroidism, and vitamin D toxicosis are much less likely in this patient.

Mild hyperproteinemia, due to hyperalbuminemia, is due to dehydration.

Hyponatremia and high normal potassium should cause suspicion of Addison's disease. While these electrolyte abnormalities are not marked, and result in a Na:K ratio of 24, they should prompt an ACTH stimulation test. Hyponatremia and hyperkalemia in this patient, on the other hand, could be a result of renal disease. Hypochloridemia is consistent with hyponatremia. Low total CO_2 is consistent with metabolic acidosis, and the anion gap is increased due to increased unmeasured anions, which in this dehydrated hypovolemic patient are probably lactic acids.

Mild increase in serum amylase and lipase activities are probably secondary to decreased glomerular filtration.

Endocrine Data

The immeasurably low cortisol concentration with a "flat-line" response to ACTH confirms hypoadrenocorticism

Summary

Hypoadrenocorticism

CASE 50

Signalment: 11-year-old spayed female beagle
History: Polyuria, polydipsia, polyphagia, and bilateral symmetrical alopecia for 5 months
Physical Examination: "Pot-bellied," comedones in inguinal region, panting

Hematology		Reference Range
PCV (%)	50	37–55
NCC (×10³/μl)	**22.6**	6–17
Segs (×10³/μl)	**20.0**	3–11.5
Monos (×10³/μl)	**2.3**	0.1–1.3
Lymphs (×10³/μl)	**0**	1–4.8
Eos (×10³/μl)	0	0.1–1.2
NRBC (×10³/μl)	**0.3**	0
Platelets (×10³/μl)	Adequate	200–500
TP (P) (g/dl)	7.6	6–8

Biochemical Profile		Reference Range
Gluc (mg/dl)	**140 (7.7)**	65–122 (3.5–6.7 mmol/L)
BUN (mg/dl)	**6 (2.1)**	7–28 (2.5–10.0 mmol/L)
Creat (mg/dl)	1.0	0.9–1.7
Ca (mg/dl)	10.2	9.0–11.2
Phos (mg/dl)	**2.7 (0.9)**	2.8–6.1 (0.9–2.0)
TP (g/dl)	7.2	5.4–7.4
Alb (g/dl)	4.1	2.7–4.5
Glob (g/dl)	3.1	1.9–3.4
T. Bili (mg/dl)	0.2	0–0.4
Chol (mg/dl)	**460 (12.0)**	130–370 (3.4–9.6)
ALT (IU/L)	**400**	10–120
ALP (IU/L)	**4500**	35–280
Na (mEq/L)	**159**	145–158
K (mEq/L)	**3.9**	4.1–5.5
CL (mEq/L)	127	106–127
TCO₂ (mEq/L)	20	14–27
An. gap (mEq/L)	16	8–25

Urinalysis	
Specific Gravity	**1.005**

Endocrine Data		Reference Range
ACTH stimulation		
serum cortisol (μg/dl)(pre)	**12 (331)**	1–4 (28–110)
serum cortisol (μg/dl)(post)	15.5	<20
Low dose dexamethasone suppression test		
serum cortisol (μg/dl)(pre)	**9.0 (248)**	1–4 (28–110)
serum cortisol (μg/dl)(3 hour post)	**8.0 (221)**	<1.5 (41)
serum cortisol (μg/dl)(8 hour post)	**6.0 (166)**	<1.5 (41)
High dose dexamethasone suppression test		
serum cortisol (μg/dl)(Pre)	**10 (276)**	1–4 (28–110)
serum cortisol (μg/dl)(post)	**8 (221)**	<1.5 (41)
endogenous ACTH (pg/ml)	**10 (2.2)**	20–100 (4.4–22.0)

Interpretive Discussion

Hematology

Mature neutrophilia, monocytosis, and lymphopenia are typically seen with increased endogenous or exogenous corticosteroids. Increased concentration of nucleated RBCs are seen with a variety of conditions; in this case they are likely secondary to hyperadrenocorticism.

Biochemical Profile

Mild hyperglycemia is consistent with increased endogenous or exogenous corticosteroids. Glucocorticoids increase gluconeogenesis and decrease peripheral utilization of glucose by antagonizing the effects of insulin.

The BUN concentration is below the reference range. While decreased BUN may be associated with liver failure or inadequate protein intake, diuresis will also result in increased urinary loss of urea nitrogen. In this case, diuresis is probably stimulated by glucocorticoids.

Hypercholesterolemia is associated with numerous conditions, including hypothyroidism, diabetes mellitus, hyperadrenocorticism, and cholestasis. In this patient, the increase is probably due to hyperadrenocorticism.

Alanine aminotransferase activity is mildly increased, indicating glucocorticoid-induced increase in ALT production or hepatocellular damage. Hepatocellular damage is an important feature of steroid hepatopathy, which may be occurring in this dog. Alkaline phosphatase activity is markedly increased. While cholestasis may result in an increase of this magnitude, bilirubin is not increased, suggesting that the increase is likely due to corticosteroid induction of alkaline phosphatase. Activities of this magnitude are almost always related to steroid effect. Determination of steroid-induced alkaline phosphatase isoenzyme would be helpful.

Mild hypernatremia and hypokalemia are commonly seen in approximately 50% of dogs with hyperadrenocorticism.

Urinalysis

Urine specific gravity is low, and is likely due to hyperadrenocorticism. Glucocorticoids are thought to interfere with ADH receptors, resulting in isosthenuria or hyposthenuria, and polyuria and polydipsia.

Endocrine Data

ACTH stimulation: The baseline cortisol concentration is well above normal and the post-stimulation cortisol concentration is within the reference range. While most dogs with hyperadrenocorticism have normal basal cortisol concentrations, this increase is very suggestive of hyperadrenocorticism. While dogs with pituitary dependent hyperplasia (PDH) have hyperplastic adrenals and dogs with functional adrenocortical tumors have the potential to respond to ACTH stimulation by increasing cortisol production and release, not all do so. Cortisol increases above the reference range following ACTH stimulation in approximately 85% of dogs with pituitary dependent disease, and in approximately 50% of dogs with adrenal tumors. In summary, while ACTH stimulation is a useful screening test for PDH and adrenal tumors, cortisol concentrations do not exceed the high end of the reference range in many dogs. Thus, this dog may have pituitary dependent disease or an adrenal tumor, based on the ACTH stimulation results.

Low and High Dose Dexamethasone Suppression: Dexamethasone screening tests are diagnostically useful because in patients with pituitary dependent disease, the abnormal pituitary is somewhat resistant to the negative feedback action of cortisol. Moreover, while dexamethasone may inhibit endogenous ACTH production in dogs with adrenal tumors, endogenous ACTH production is probably already maximally suppressed, and at any rate, these tumors usually autonomously secrete cortisol, independent of ACTH. In normal dogs, endogenous ACTH is suppressed by dexamethasone, resulting in a rapid decline in plasma cortisol concentrations which remain suppressed for up to 48 hours. Thus, since this dog's cortisol concentration did not decrease, either pituitary dependent disease resulting in adrenocortical hyperplasia, or adrenal neoplasia, is present.

Endogenous ACTH: Endogenous ACTH is below the reference range in this dog, indicating that the dog has a functional adrenal tumor, rather than pituitary disease.

Summary

Hyperadrenocorticism due to functional adrenal tumor. On abdominal radiographs, a calcified mass cranial to the right kidney was observed. On ultrasound examination, a large right adrenal mass was seen. The left adrenal was not detectable. A CT scan of the brain was normal.

CASE 51

Signalment: 4-year-old MC Golden Retriever
History: Polyuria, polydipsia for several months, on medication for flea allergy dermatitis
Physical Examination: Exudative, erythematous plaques in inguinal area, "pot-bellied" appearance

Hematology		Reference Range
PCV (%)	40	37–55
NCC (×10³/µl)	**25.9**	6–17
Segs (×10³/µl)	**23.4**	3–11.5
Monos (×10³/µl)	**2.0**	0.1–1.3
Lymphs (×10³/µl)	**0.4**	1–4.8
Eos (×10³/µl)	0.1	0.1–1.2
Platelets (×10³/µl)	Adequate	200–500
TP (P) (g/dl)	7.5	6–8

Biochemical Profile		Reference Range
Gluc (mg/dl)	**140 (7.7)**	65–122 (3.5–6.7 mmol/L)
BUN (mg/dl)	18	7–28
Creat (mg/dl)	1.2	0.9–1.7
Ca (mg/dl)	10.5	9.0–11.2
Phos (mg/dl)	4.0	2.8–6.1
TP (g/dl)	7.0	5.4–7.4
Alb (g/dl)	4.0	2.7–4.5
Glob (g/dl)	3.0	1.9–3.4
T. Bili (mg/dl)	0.2	0–0.4
Chol (mg/dl)	350	130–370
ALT (IU/L)	110	10–120
AST (IU/L)	30	16–40
ALP (IU/L)	**5500**	35–280
GGT (IU/L)	**260**	0–6
Na (mEq/L)	148	145–158
K (mEq/L)	5.0	4.1–5.5
CL (mEq/L)	112	106–127
TCO₂ (mEq/L)	16	14–27
An. gap (mEq/L)	25	8–25

Urinalysis			
Color	Yellow	**Urine Sediment**	
Transparency	Cloudy	WBCs/hpf	2
Sp. Gr.	**1.002**	RBCs/hpf	2
Protein	Negative	Epith cells/hpf	0
Gluc	Negative	Casts/lpf	0
Bilirubin	Negative	Crystals	0
Blood	Negative	Bacteria	4+
pH	6.5		

Endocrine Data		Reference Range
ACTH stimulation		
serum cortisol (µg/dl)(pre)	1.2	1–4
serum cortisol (µg/dl)(post)	**1.2 (33)**	>10.5; <20 (>290; <550 nmol/L)
Low dose dexamethasone suppression test		
serum cortisol (µg/dl)(pre)	2.0	1–4
serum cortisol (µg/dl)(3-hour post)	**2.0 (55)**	<1.5 (<41nmol/L)
serum cortisol (µg/dl)(8-hour post)	**1.7 (47)**	<1.5 (<41nmol/L)

Interpretive Discussion

Hematology

Mature neutrophilia, monocytosis, and lymphopenia are indicative of a corticosteroid (stress) leukogram.

Biochemical Profile

Mild hyperglycemia is consistent with increased endogenous or exogenous corticosteroids.

Alkaline phosphatase activity is markedly increased. While cholestasis may result in an increase of this magnitude, bilirubin is not increased, suggesting that the increase is likely due to corticosteroid induction of alkaline phosphatase. Determination of steroid-induced alkaline phosphatase isoenzyme would be helpful.

Gamma glutamyl transferase activity is also markedly increased, and with the lack of increase in ALT and AST activities, as well as bilirubin concentration, corticosteroid induction is likely.

The combination of mild hyperglycemia and increased ALP and GGT activities, with no other evidence of cholestasis, should trigger further endocrine testing.

Urinalysis

Low urine specific gravity (often hyposthenuria) is commonly seen in patients with hyperadrenocorticism. Glucocorticoids are thought to interfere with ADH receptors, resulting in isosthenuria or hyposthenuria, and polyuria and polydipsia. Bacteriuria without significant pyuria may also occur with hyperadrenocorticism.

Endocrine Data

ACTH stimulation: Patients with iatrogenic hyperadrenocorticism have a "flat-line" response to ACTH stimulation (much like a patient with hypoadrenocorticism) due to feedback to the pituitary and secondary adrenal atrophy. While some corticosteroid drugs cross-react on the cortisol assay, the post-ACTH response will not be higher than the pre-ACTH response.

Low Dose Dexamethasone Suppression: LDDS is not helpful in diagnosing iatrogenic hyperadrenocorticism. The pituitary is already responding to feedback from iatrogenic corticosteroids, and adrenal glands are atrophied.

Summary

Iatrogenic Cushing disease which resulted from Vetalog injections for flea allergy dermatitis. Fleas were eliminated, and the dog was slowly withdrawn from corticosteroids by treating on alternate days with decreasing doses over several months.

CASE 52

Signalment: 10-year-old spayed female Airedale
History: "Leaking" urine, polydipsia, limping
Physical Examination: Ruptured anterior cruciate ligament, "pot-bellied," mild truncal alopecia

Hematology		Reference Range
PCV (%)	58	37–55
NCC (×10³/μl)	24.4	6–17
Segs (×10³/μl)	21.5	3–11.5
Monos (×10³/μl)	2.4	0.1–1.3
Lymphs (×10³/μl)	0	1–4.8
NRBC (×10³/μl)	0.5	0
Platelets (×10³/μl)	Adequate	200–500

Biochemical Profile		Reference Range
Gluc (mg/dl)	130 (7.1)	65–122 (3.5–6.7 mmol/L)
BUN (mg/dl)	18	7–28
Creat (mg/dl)	1.2	0.9–1.7
Ca (mg/dl)	10.2	9.0–11.2
Phos (mg/dl)	4.9	2.8–6.1
TP (g/dl)	5.7	5.4–7.4
Alb (g/dl)	2.7	2.7–4.5
Glob (g/dl)	3.0	1.9–3.4
T. Bili	0.3	0–0.4
Chol (mg/dl)	350	130–370
ALT (IU/L)	65	10–120
AST (IU/L)	60	16–40
ALP (IU/L)	4000	35–280

Urinalysis	
Sp. Gr.	1.008
Bacteria	Many

Endocrine Data		Reference Range
ACTH stimulation:		
serum cortisol (μg/dl)(pre)	8 (221)	1–4 (28–110 nmol/L)
serum cortisol (μg/dl)(post)	20 (552)	<20 (<552 nmol/L)
Low dose dexamethasone suppression test		
serum cortisol (μg/dl)(pre)	6 (166)	1–4 (28–110 nmol/L)
serum cortisol (μg/dl)(3-hour post)	0.9	<1.5
serum cortisol (μg/dl)(8-hour post)	1.7 (47)	<1.5 (<41nmol/L)
High dose dexamethasone suppression test		
serum cortisol (μg/dl)(Pre)	9 (248)	1–4 (28–110 nmol/L)
serum cortisol (μg/dl)(post)	3 (83)	<1.5 (<41nmol/L)
endogenous ACTH (pg/ml)	350 (77)	20–100 (4.4–22.0 pmol/L)

Interpretive Discussion

Hematology

The PCV is mildly increased, with increased nucleated erythrocyte concentration. Possibilities for this combination might include hypoxia or other causes of increased erythropoietin concentration. Dogs with hyperadrenocorticism will sometimes have increased erythropoiesis. Additionally, corticosteroids may inhibit removal of NRBC by macrophages in spleen. Mature neutrophilia, monoctosis, and lymphopenia are indicative of a stress leukogram.

Biochemical Profile

Mild hyperglycemia is consistent with a stress leukogram, and may be a result of increased endogenous or exogenous glucocorticoids.

Alkaline phosphatase is markedly increased, AST is mildly increased, and cholesterol is borderline high. No other abnormalities are present. Increased alkaline phosphatase activity and mild hypercholesterolemia may be secondary to cholestasis; however, serum bilirubin is not increased. Alkaline phosphatase activity may also increase secondary to steroid induction. This is most likely given the magnitude of increase. The slight increase in serum AST activity may be due to mild steroid hepatopathy or steroid induction.

Urinalysis

Urine specific gravity is quite low, and while it is not necessarily abnormal, it is consistent with decreased urinary concentrating ability in dogs with hyperadrenocorticism, related to decreased responsiveness to ADH. Bacteriuria without pyuria may be seen in dogs with hyperadrenocorticism.

Physical exam, history, stress leukogram, hyperglycemia, and increased serum alkaline phosphatase activity should trigger screening tests for hyperadrenocorticism.

Endocrine Data

ACTH stimulation: Baseline cortisol is above normal and poststimulation is "borderline." Stimulation of above 20 is consistent with hyperadrenocorticism. Eighty-five percent of dogs with pituitary dependent hyperplasia stimulate, as do approximately 50% of dogs with adrenal tumors. Thus, the ACTH stimulation is not diagnostic in this dog, but is suspicious.

Low dose dexamethasone suppression: Baseline cortisol is above normal. The dog suppressed at 3 hours, with escape from suppression at 8 hours. In normal dogs, endogenous ACTH is suppressed by dexamethasone, resulting in a rapid decline in plasma cortisol concentrations which remain suppressed for up to 48 hours. Most dogs with adrenal tumors show no suppression at 3 or 8 hours. If a dog suppresses at 3 hours, but does not remain suppressed at 8 hours, it is likely that the dog has PDH, rather than an adrenal tumor. This "escape" is thought to be due to rapid clearance of dexamethasone.

High dose dexamethasone suppression: Baseline cortisol is above normal. The dog did not suppress to the range for normal dogs. Dogs with adrenal disease do not suppress, and most dogs with pituitary dependent adrenal hyperplasia (PPH) do suppress. Very high dose steroids will suppress ACTH production, and hence cortisol secretion, even with PPD. However, most dogs with pituitary macroadenomas do not suppress; an endogenous ACTH serum concentration is indicated.

Endogenous ACTH: Dogs with PDH have normal to increased endogenous ACTH, while dogs with adrenal tumors have decreased endogenous ACTH. Thus, this dog has pituitary dependent disease.

Summary

A large pituitary macroadenoma was present in this dog. Note that multiple endocrine tests were required to make this diagnosis.

CASE 53

Signalment: 8-month-old intact male dog
History: Suddenly collapsed during grooming. Bloody diarrhea.
Physical Examination: Extreme weakness, bradycardia, and cool extremities.

Hematology		Reference Range
PCV (%)	42	37–55
Hgb (g/dl)	13.3	12–18
RBC (×10⁶/µl)	6.6	5.5–8.5
MCV (fl)	64	60–72
MCHC (g/dl)	32	34–38
NCC (×10³/µl)	12.0	6–17
Segs (×10³/µl)	7.2	3–11.5
Monos (×10³/µl)	0.6	0.1–1.3
Lymphs (×10³/µl)	3.6	1–4.8
Eos (×10³/µl)	0.6	0.1–1.2
Platelets (×10³/µl)	410	200–500
TP (P) (g/dl)	6.9	6–8
Hemopathology: Normal		

Biochemical Profile		Reference Range
Gluc (mg/dl)	87	65–122
BUN (mg/dl)	**63 (22.5)**	7–28 (2.5–10.0 mmol/L)
Creat (mg/dl)	1.6	0.9–1.7
Ca (mg/dl)	10.3	9.0–11.2
Phos (mg/dl)	5.6	2.8–6.1
TP (g/dl)	6.8	5.4–7.4
Alb (g/dl)	3.9	2.7–4.5
Glob (g/dl)	2.9	1.9–3.4
T. Bili (mg/dl)	0.3	0–0.4
Chol (mg/dl)	230	130–370
ALT (IU/L)	80	10–120
AST (IU/L)	32	16–40
ALP (IU/L)	90	35–280
Na (mEq/L)	**127**	145–158
K (mEq/L)	**7.5**	4.1–5.5
CL (mEq/L)	**99**	106–127
TCO₂ (mEq/L)	**12**	14–27
An. gap (mEq/L)	23	8–25

Urinalysis			
Color	Yellow	**Urine Sediment**	
Transparency	Clear	WBCs/hpf	0–1
Sp. Gr.	**1.019**	RBCs/hpf	2–3
Protein	Negative	Epith cells/hpf	1–2 transitional
Gluc	Negative	Casts/lpf	0
Bilirubin	Negative	Crystals	0
Blood	Negative	Bacteria	0
pH	6.0		

Endocrine Data		Reference Range
ACTH stimulation:		
serum cortisol (µg/dl)(pre)	1.1	1–4
serum cortisol (µg/dl)(post)	**1.3 (36)**	10–20 (276–552 nmol/L)

Interpretive Discussion

Hematology

The CBC reveals no significant abnormalities.

Biochemical Profile

This dog is azotemic. Since urine concentration is not adequate (i.e., it is not >1.030), this may be a renal azotemia, but prerenal azotemia with inadequate renal concentrating ability may occur in hypoadrenocorticism. The hypotension and dehydration that accompany hypoadrenocortism may result in azotemia while hyponatremia and solute diuresis may result in medullary washout which, in turn, limits renal concentrating ability. The result is azotemia with a urine specific gravity indicating inadequate renal concentrating ability.

Hyponatremia and hyperkalemia, in combination with the abnormal response to ACTH stimulation, confirms the diagnosis of hypoadrenocorticism (see discussion of the ACTH stimulation test below). While a Na/K ratio <23:1 is suggestive of hypoadrenocorticism, hyponatremia and hyperkalemia are not specific for this disease. Oliguric or anuric renal failure are common causes of hyponatremia and hyperkalemia and should be considered when these abnormalities are observed, but the response to ACTH stimulation should be adequate to distinguish these diseases.

Hypochloremia is common in animals with hypoadrenocorticism. In renal tubules, Cl is reabsorbed with Na in both the proximal tubule and the loop of Henle. After hyponatremia develops, the concentration of Na in the ultrafiltrate is decreased, and this, in turn, decreases the amount of Na available for reabsorption in these portions of the nephron. The decreased Na absorption results in decreased Cl absorption and hypochloremia.

Decreased serum total CO_2 concentration suggests metabolic acidosis. Metabolic acidosis is common in hypoadrenocorticism and results from decreased tissue perfusion secondary to hypotension and from decreased renal tubular excretion of H+ secondary to mineralocorticoid deficiency.

Urinalysis

Except for the evidence of inadequate urine concentrating ability (see the discussion of azotemia above), the urinalysis is normal.

Endocrine Data

The inadequate response to ACTH stimulation in combination with hyponatremia and hyperkalemia confirms hypoadrenocorticism. Dogs with hypoadrenocorticism commonly have decreased basal plasma cortisol concentrations which fail to increase or increase only slightly after ACTH stimulation. If these values do increase after ACTH stimulation, they are usually well below normal post-ACTH stimulation values, especially in dogs with primary hypoadrenocorticism.

Summary

Hyponatremia, hyperkalemia, and a Na:K ratio of 17:1 suggest hypoadrenocorticism. An inadequate response to ACTH stimulation confirms this disease. The azotemia with evidence of inadequate urine concentrating ability, while typical of primary renal failure, is more likely due to a combination of prerenal azotemia and decreased renal concentrating ability resulting from the effects of mineralocorticoid deficiency. It is typical of ill animals to have a stress leukogram (lymphopenia); absence of stress leukogram in this ill animal is compatible with hypoadrenocorticism.

CASE 54

Signalment: 6-year-old male dog

History: Change in temperament from docile to irritable. Severe constipation for several days.

Physical Examination: No abnormalities detected

Hematology		Reference Range
PCV (%)	44	37–55
Hgb (g/dl)	14.5	12–18
RBC (×10⁶/µl)	6.7	5.5–8.5
MCV (fl)	66	60–72
MCHC (g/dl)	33	34–38
NCC (×10³/µl)	15.6	6–17
Segs (×10³/µl)	**12.7**	3–11.5
Monos (×10³/µl)	0.2	0.1–1.3
Lymphs (×10³/µl)	2.4	1–4.8
Eos (×10³/µl)	0.3	0.1–1.2
Platelets (×10³/µl)	440	200–500
TP (P) (g/dl)	6.8	6–8
Hemopathology: Normal		

Biochemical Profile		Reference Range
Gluc (mg/dl)	80	65–122
BUN (mg/dl)	28	7–28
Creat (mg/dl)	1.5	0.9–1.7
Ca (mg/dl)	**14.3 (3.57)**	9.0–11.2 (2.25–2.80 mmol/L)
Phos (mg/dl)	**1.7 (0.5)**	2.8–6.1 (0.9–2.0 mmol/L)
TP (g/dl)	6.1	5.4–7.4
Alb (g/dl)	3.4	2.7–4.5
Glob (g/dl)	2.7	1.9–3.4
T. Bili (mg/dl)	0.4	0–0.4
Chol (mg/dl)	235	130–370
ALT (IU/L)	100	10–120
AST (IU/L)	33	16–40
ALP (IU/L)	**285**	35–280
Na (mEq/L)	145	145–158
K (mEq/L)	5.3	4.1–5.5
CL (mEq/L)	115	106–127
TCO₂ (mEq/L)	21	14–27
An. gap (mEq/L)	14	8–25

Urinalysis (catheterized)			
Color	Yellow	**Urine Sediment**	
Transparency	Clear	WBCs/hpf	0–2
Sp. Gr.	**1.011**	RBCs/hpf	0
Protein	Negative	Epith cells/hpf	0
Gluc	Negative	Casts/lpf	0
Bilirubin	Negative	Crystals	0
Blood	Negative	Bacteria	0
pH	6.5		

Endocrine Data		Reference Range
Intact parathormone	**22**	2–13 (pmol/L)
PTHrp	Undetectable	<0.2 (pmol/L)

Interpretive Discussion

Hematology

In light of normal results for other erythrocyte measurements, the decreased MCHC is marginal and not important.

The mild mature neutrophilia, in the absence of lymphopenia, suggests normal variability or an epinephrine-mediated response. This dog's irritability may have predisposed it to epinephrine release when the venipuncture was performed.

Biochemical Profile

Hypercalcemia and hypophosphatemia can occur with primary hyperparathyroidism and pseudohyperparathyroidism (hypercalcemia of malignancy). In this case, the increased intact parathormone (iPTH) and normal parathormone-related protein (PTHrp) concentrations are most suggestive of primary hyperparathyroidism (see discussion of hormone assays below). Other causes of hypercalcemia include vitamin D toxicosis, excessive bone resorption, and renal failure (5–10% of these cases in dogs), but serum phosphorus concentration is typically normal to increased in these cases.

The slightly increased serum alkaline phosphatase activity is not significant. There is no evidence suggesting either cholestasis or increased corticosteroid levels. Since this dog has an abnormality of calcium and phosphorus metabolism, it is possible that altered bone metabolism is occurring. Although the net effect in this animal is probably bone demineralization, increased osteoblastic activity, as part of effort to regenerate bone, may have resulted in this slight increase in activity.

Urinalysis

Low urine specific gravity may reflect this dog's hydration status and, therefore, may be normal in this patient. Hypercalcemia can, however, interfere with renal concentrating ability and can result in decreased urine specific gravity with subsequent polyuria and polydipsia. Nephrocalcinosis, other toxic effects of calcium on renal tubules, and interference with the action of antidiuretic hormone are possible mechanisms for decreased concentrating ability in hypercalcemic animals. The absence of polyuria and polydipsia in this dog suggests that calcium interference with renal concentrating ability is not a major factor.

Endocrine Data

Increased intact parathormone (iPTH) concentration and undetectable PTH-related protein (PTHrp) concentration indicate that this dog has primary hyperparathyroidism, rather than pseudohyperparathyroidism. The iPTH concentrations are increased due to overproduction of PTH by hyperplastic or neoplastic parathyroid glands. Parathormone-related protein is synthesized by malignant cells of neoplasms such as lymphoma and apocrine gland adenocarcinoma of the anal sac, but not by the parathyroid glands, and concentrations of PTHrp are, therefore, not increased in animals with primary hyperparathyroidism.

Summary

The combination of hypercalcemia, hypophosphatemia, increased iPTH concentration, and undetectable PTHrp concentration indicate primary hyperparathyroidism in this case. A mass in the neck region compatible in location with the parathyroid gland was found during a more thorough physical examination. Surgical removal and histopathologic examination revealed a parathyroid adenoma. This dog's clinical signs and serum calcium and phosphorus concentrations returned to normal after surgery. Irritability is unusual in hypercalcemic dogs; dullness is more common.

CASE 55

Signalment: 9-year-old intact male dog
History: One seizure. Occasional tremors observed.
Physical Examination: Physical abnormalities, but had seizure during examination.

Hematology		Reference Range
PCV (%)	44	37–55
Hgb (g/dl)	15.2	12–18
RBC (×10⁶/µl)	7.1	5.5–8.5
MCV (fl)	62	60–72
MCHC (g/dl)	35	34–38
NCC (×10³/µl)	**20.2**	6–17
Segs (×10³/µl)	**17.2**	3–11.5
Monos (×10³/µl)	**2.4**	0.1–1.3
Lymphs (×10³/µl)	**0.6**	1–4.8
Platelets (×10³/µl)	470	200–500
TP (P) (g/dl)	7.2	6–8
Hemopathology: Normal		

Biochemical Profile		Reference Range
Gluc (mg/dl)	**138 (7.6)**	65–122 (3.5–6.7 mmol/L)
BUN (mg/dl)	14	7–28
Creat (mg/dl)	**0.5**	0.9–1.7
Ca (mg/dl)	**4.0 (1.0)**	9.0–11.2 (2.25–2.80 mmol/L)
Phos (mg/dl)	**7.0 (2.3)**	2.8–6.1 (0.9–2.9 mmol/L)
TP (g/dl)	7.0	5.4–7.4
Alb (g/dl)	3.6	2.7–4.5
Glob (g/dl)	3.4	1.9–3.4
T. Bili (mg/dl)	0.4	0–0.4
Chol (mg/dl)	161	130–370
ALT (IU/L)	38	10–120
AST (IU/L)	18	16–40
ALP (IU/L)	176	35–280
Na (mEq/L)	145	145–158
K (mEq/L)	4.4	4.1–5.5
CL (mEq/L)	**103**	106–127
TCO₂ (mEq/L)	22	14–27
An. gap (mEq/L)	24	8–25

Urinalysis			
Color	Yellow	**Urine Sediment**	
Transparency	Clear	WBCs/hpf	0
Sp. Gr.	1.032	RBCs/hpf	0
Protein	Negative	Epith cells/hpf	0
Gluc	Negative	Casts/lpf	0
Bilirubin	Trace	Crystals	0
Blood	Negative	Bacteria	0
pH	6.0		

Endocrine Data		Reference Range
iPTH (pmol/L)	**2**	2–13

Interpretive Discussion

Hematology

Mature neutrophilia, lymphopenia, and monocytosis are typical of a stress leukogram.

Biochemical Profile

The serum glucose concentration is in the range typical for glucocorticoid-induced hyperglycemia. Stress is the most likely cause in this case, particularly in light of the leukogram.

Decreased serum creatinine concentration is meaningless in most cases. This abnormality can result from diuresis, but, if this is the cause, the BUN concentration is usually also decreased. The absence of a history of polyuria and the normal BUN concentration make diuresis unlikely in this case.

Hypocalcemia and hyperphosphatemia can occur in renal failure, pancreatitis with prerenal azotemia, eating a diet containing excessive phosphorus, or hypoparathyroidism. Hypoparathyroidism is most likely in this case. Normal BUN concentration and decreased serum creatinine concentration indicate that renal function is normal. Clinical signs are not typical of pancreatitis, and there is no evidence of a prerenal azotemia. This dog may be receiving a diet with excessive phosphorus, but this is very unlikely if the dog is receiving a commercial diet. Hypoalbuminemia is another cause of hypocalcemia, but the absence of hypoalbuminemia indicates that this is not a consideration. Vitamin D deficiency may also result in hypocalcemia, but hypophosphatemia rather than hyperphosphatemia is typical of such a deficiency. Hypoparathyroidism can be confirmed by measuring the serum intact parathormone concentration (see below).

Slight hypochloremia, in the absence of abnormalities in Na, K, or total CO_2, is probably insignificant.

Urinalysis

The urinalysis is normal.

Endocrine Data

The serum intact parathormone (iPTH) concentration is at the bottom of the reference range. The normal response of the parathyroid glands to hypocalcemia is production of PTH. Low normal iPTH concentration in a hypocalcemic animal strongly suggests inability of the parathyroid glands to respond to hypocalcemia and, therefore, hypoparathyroidism. Other possible causes of hypocalcemia (discussed above) should result in high normal to increased iPTH concentrations.

Summary

The combination of hypocalcemia with low normal iPTH concentration indicate hypoparathyroidism. Other diseases can result in hypocalcemia and hyperphosphatemia, but iPTH concentration in these diseases is typically high normal to increased.

CASE 56

Signalment: 13-year-old MC dog
History: Polyuria, frequent urination with small volumes
Physical Examination: Overweight

Hematology		Reference Range
PCV (%)	**36.0**	37–55
Hgb (g/dl)	13.4	12–18
RBC (×10⁶/µl)	**5.26**	5.5–8.5
MCV (fl)	69.0	60–72
MCHC (g/dl)	37.0	34–38
NCC(×10³/µl)	**18.1**	6–17
Segs (×10³/µl)	**16.7**	3–11.5
Monos (×10³/µl)	1.3	0.1–1.3
Lymphs (×10³/µl)	**0.2**	1.0–4.8
Platelets (×10³/µl)	452	200–500
TP (P) (g/dl)	**8.2**	6–8

Hemopathology: few Howell-Jolly bodies

Biochemical Profile		Reference Range
Gluc (mg/dl)	**806 (44.3)**	65–122 (3.5–6.7 mmol/L)
BUN (mg/dl)	**81 (28.9)**	7–28 (2.5–10.0 mmol/L)
Creat (mg/dl)	1.6	0.9–1.7
Ca (mg/dl)	**8.4 (2.1)**	9.0–11.2 (2.25–2.80 mmol/L)
ionized Ca++ (mg/dl)	**3.56**	4.5–5.6
Phos (mg/dl)	**7.2 (2.3)**	2.8–6.1 (0.9–2.0 mmol/L)
TP (g/dl)	6.0	5.4–7.4
Alb (g/dl)	3.3	2.7–4.5
Glob (g/dl)	2.7	1.9–3.4
T. Bili (mg/dl)	**1.3 (22.2)**	0–0.4 (0–6.8 µmol/L)
Chol (mg/dl)	**467 (12.1)**	130–370 (3.4–9.6 mmol/L)
ALT (IU/L)	**1355**	0–120
AST (IU/L)	**341**	16–40
ALP (IU/L)	**4660**	35–280
GGT (IU/L)	**373**	0–6
CK (IU/L)	**266**	50–250
Na (mEq/L)	**144**	145–158
K (mEq/L)	**3.8**	4.1–5.5
CL (mEq/L)	**98**	106–127
TCO₂ (mEq/L)	18.5	14–27
An. gap (mEq/L)	**31.3**	8–25
Amylase (IU/L)	**1687**	50–1250
Lipase (IU/L)	**3746**	30–560

Urinalysis			
Color	Yellow	**Urine Sediment**	
Transparency	Cloudy	WBCs/hpf	**50–100**
Sp. Gr.	**1.014**	RBCs/hpf	**>100**
Protein	**2+**	Epith cells/hpf	Negative
Gluc	**4+**	Casts/lpf	Negative
Bilirubin	Negative	Crystals	Negative
Blood	**4+**	Bacteria	**3+ rods**
pH	5.0		
ketones	Negative		

Coagulation Data		Reference Range
PT (sec)	7.5	7.5–10.5
aPPT (seconds)	**18.2**	10.5–16.5
FDPs (µg/ml)	**1:12**	<1:10

Endocrine Data		Reference Range
Free T4 (ng/dl)	**<0.15**	1.2–3.4
total T4 (µg/dl)	**0.85**	1.5–3.5
endog TSH (ng/ml)	**0.05**	0.1–0.45

Interpretive Discussion

Hematology

The PCV and total RBC count are marginally decreased, with no abnormalities in red blood cell size, hemoglobin content, or morphology. One should consider recent blood loss (particularly GI hemorrhage) even though plasma protein concentration is normal. Alternatively, there may be a mild normochromic, normocytic anemia associated with renal failure. The leukocyte count is increased, with a mature neutrophilia and lymphopenia. This is a stress leukogram, and may support the possibility of hyperadrenocorticism as part of the disease process.

Biochemical Profile

The serum glucose concentration is markedly increased. This is beyond the level encountered due to excitement (sympathetic activation) or stress (glucocorticoid release), and should immediately suggest diabetes mellitus.

The BUN is disproportionately increased relative to the mild increase in serum creatinine concentration. The BUN:creatinine ratio is 50.6, which should suggest gastrointestinal hemorrhage, leading to an increase in hepatic urea production. Nevertheless, some degree of azotemia (prerenal, renal, or postrenal) is probably also present (refer to discussion of urinalysis below). The serum phosphorus is moderately increased, and may be associated with the impaired glomerular filtration and the azotemia. Because the serum total calcium concentration is also decreased, one should consider dietary imbalance or renal disease, as causes of secondary hyperparathyroidism. See discussion of ionized Ca below.

The serum total protein and albumin concentrations are normal. Unless there is a concomitant cause for hypoproteinemia, the absence of hyperproteinemia decreases the probability for hemoconcentration and prerenal azotemia due to dehydration.

The serum cholesterol is moderately increased. This may be related to cholestasis, as indicated by the moderate increase in serum total bilirubin concentration and serum ALP and GGT activities. However, the degree of increase in cholesterol is sufficient to warrant consideration of abnormalities in lipoprotein metabolism owing to hepatic disease or an endocrine abnormality. Likewise, the degree of increase in ALP and GGT activities suggests other means for their induction beyond cholestasis, such as hyperadrenocorticism. Marked increases in serum ALT and AST activities indicate hepatocellular damage, which may have contributed to the increases in ALP and GGT activities. The serum CK activity is essentially normal, and rules out the potential contribution of muscle damage to serum AST and ALT increases. Hepatic lipidosis associated with diabetes should be considered as a cause of hepatocellular injury and cholestasis.

A marginal increase in serum amylase and marked increase in serum lipase activities may indicate the presence of pancreatitis. However, concurrent azotemia may impair renal extraction of these enzymes from the serum, leading to increases in their activities.

Serum Na, K, and Cl concentrations are decreased. One should consider typical causes for electrolyte depletion, including pathologic losses from the gastrointestinal and urinary systems, as well as a shift to third space. The marked hyperglycemia should initiate consideration of diabetic ketoacidosis with subsequent urinary electrolyte loss. However, although the anion gap is increased, the serum total CO_2 is normal. It is possible that there are concurrent causes for metabolic acidosis (ketoacidosis) and metabolic alkalosis (vomiting and/or gastrointestinal stasis).

Urinalysis

The urinary specific gravity is in the isosthenuric range, despite azotemia and hyperphosphatemia. This may be the result of renal disease, or impaired concentrating ability due to electrolyte depletion and loss of the medullary concentration gradient. There is significant proteinuria, pyuria, hematuria, and bacteriuria which most likely indicate a bacterial infection and inflammatory response in the urinary tract. In the absence of tubular casts or information regarding enzymuria or urinary fractional excretion of electrolytes, it is difficult to specify the anatomic location of this disorder. There is significant glucosuria corresponding to the marked hyperglycemia noted earlier. The absence of ketones on the dipstick speaks against the possibility of prominent ketoacidosis (and ketonuria) noted above. However, this test does not detectg one of the ketones, β-hydroxybutyric acid. However, it is anticipated that detectable ketosis will develop if untreated.

Coagulation Data

The coagulation profile indicates a slightly prolonged APTT and mildly increased FDP concentration. This may be the result of liver disease (although one may expect a change in PT prior to one in the APTT), or incipient DIC (although platelet concentration is usually decreased with DIC). If liver disease was severe enough to impair coagulation factor synthesis, one would first expect to see hypoalbuminemia and/or hypocholesterolemia. It is not possible to draw conclusions with these borderline abnormalities.

Endocrine Data

Low free T4, low total T4, and low endogenous TSH are diagnostic for secondary hypothyroidism. Secondary hypothyroidism as a result of decreased endogenous TSH is commonly associated with diabetes mellitus.

Summary

Diabetes mellitus and secondary hypothyroidism.

CASE 57

Signalment: 6-year-old M canine
History: Lethargic, quit eating
Physical Examination: Depressed, weak pulse, apparent weakness

Hematology		Reference Range
PCV (%)	46.0	37–55
Hgb (g/dl)	16.2	12–18
RBC (×10⁶/µl)	7.10	5.5–8.5
MCV (fl)	65.0	60–72
MCHC (g/dl)	35.0	34–38
NCC (×10³/µl)	**20.4**	6–17
Segs (×10³/µl)	11.4	3–11.5
Monos (×10³/µl)	**1.8**	0.1–1.3
Lymphs (×10³/µl)	**5.5**	1–4.8
Eos (×10³/µl)	**1.6**	0.1–1.2
Platelets (×10³/µl)	574	200–500
TP (P) (g/dl)	**5.9**	6–8

Hemopathology: few acanthocytes, few echinocytes, few schistocytes/fragments

Biochemical Profile		Reference Range
Gluc (mg/dl)	79	65–122
BUN (mg/dl)	**95 (33.9)**	7–28 (2.5–10.0 mmol/L)
Creat (mg/dl)	**3.8 (334)**	0.9–1.7 (80–150 µmol/L)
Ca (mg/dl)	**14.3 (3.57)**	9.0–11.2 (2.25–2.80 mmol/L)
Phos (mg/dl)	**9.9 (3.2)**	2.8–6.1 (0.9–2.0 mmol/L)
TP (g/dl)	5.8	5.4–7.4
Alb (g/dl)	3.0	2.7–4.5
Glob (g/dl)	2.8	1.9–3.4
T. Bili (mg/dl)	0.3	0–0.4
Chol (mg/dl)	130	130–370
ALT (IU/L)	62	10–120
AST (IU/L)	**108**	16–40
ALP (IU/L)	38	35–280
GGT (IU/L)	3	0–6
Na (mEq/L)	**124**	145–158
K (mEq/L)	**7.1**	4.1–5.5
CL (mEq/L)	**89**	106–127
TCO₂ (mEq/L)	**10.1**	14–27
An. gap (mEq/L)	**32**	8–25
Amylase (IU/L)	**1490**	50–1250
Lipase (IU/L)	130	30–560

Blood Gas Data (arterial)		Reference Range
pH	**7.213**	7.33–7.45
PO₂ (mmHg)	101.0	67–92
PCO₂ (mmHg)	27.6	24–39
HCO₃ (mEq/L)	**10.4**	14–24
ionized Ca++ (mg/dl)	**6.40**	4.5–5.6

Urinalysis			
Color	Yellow	**Urine Sediment**	
Transparency	Cloudy	WBCs/hpf	1–4
Sp. Gr.	**1.018**	RBCs/hpf	1–2
Protein	Negative	Epith cells/hpf	1–2
Gluc	Negative	Casts/lpf	Negative
Bilirubin	Trace	Crystals	Negative
Blood	Negative	Bacteria	Negative
pH	6.0	Other	
UPC	0.93		

Endocrine Data		Reference Range
ACTH stimulation:		
serum cortisol (µg/dl) (pre)	**0.04 (1.1)**	1–4 (28–110 nmol/L)
serum cortisol (µg/dl)(post)	**0.09 (2.5)**	<20 (<552 nmol/L)

Interpretive Discussion

Hematology

There are no erythrocyte abnormalities. There is a lymphocytosis, which should prompt brief consideration of lymphoma (note the hypercalcemia), or which could be explained by a corticosteroid deficiency. Whenever an ill animal does not have a stress leukogram, one should consider the possibility of hypoadrenocorticism.

Biochemical Profile

The BUN, serum creatinine, and phosphorus concentrations are moderately increased. These findings indicate decreased glomerular filtration rate. However, one cannot differentiate the nature of the azotemia (prerenal, renal, or postrenal) based on these findings alone. Refer to the discussion of urinalysis results for further interpretation.

The serum total calcium concentration is moderately increased. The most common causes for this would be malignancy-associated hypercalcemia, hypoadrenocorticism, or renal failure. One might also consider primary hyperparathyroidism and vitamin D toxicosis.

The serum total protein, albumin, and globulin concentrations are normal. The absence of hemoconcentration decreases the probability for prerenal azotemia associated with dehydration.

There are no significant changes in indices of liver disease, with the exception of a mild increase in serum AST activity. This may be due to mild hepatocellular damage or muscle damage, but is small enough that further consideration may not be necessary.

There are significant decreases in the serum concentrations of Na and Cl, as well as a significant increase in serum K concentration. The Na:K ratio is 17.5, which is strongly suggestive of hypoadrenocorticism. The presence of a metabolic acidosis (low total CO_2) is consistent with that possibility, and the anion gap may be increased owing to accumulation of unmeasured anions such as lactic acids or phosphates.

Blood Gas Data

The blood gas data indicate an uncompensated metabolic acidosis (decreased pH and HCO_3, normal pCO_2). The ionized calcium concentration is increased, further supporting a finding of hypercalcemia. One should consider the possibilities of either primary hypoadrenocorticism or renal disease resulting in a functional deficit in response to corticosteroids and calcium retention.

Urinalysis

The urinary specific gravity reveals only marginal concentrating ability, which may result from either renal disease, or loss of the medullary concentration gradient due to electrolyte depletion. This is a common finding in hypoadrenocorticism that should prompt further diagnostics to rule out primary renal disease. The absence of nonregenerative anemia is evidence counter to chronic renal disease. The dipstick protein was negative, and the UPC is <1.0, supporting no significant urinary protein loss.

Endocrine Data

The pre and post ACTH cortisol concentrations are both low, and there is an inadequate response. This confirms hypoadrenocorticism.

Summary

Hypoadrenocorticism with typical azotemia secondary to hypovolemia. While there is no biochemical evidence of hemoconcentration, hypovolemia is a consistent event in the pathogenesis of azotemia associated with hypoadrenocorticism.